Praise for Annie Sklaver Orenstein:

"In *Always a Sibling*, Annie Sklaver Orenstein captures the raw and devastating grief of losing her brother Captain Ben Sklaver to war, and the life-changing ripple effect that comes from such a loss. Orenstein shares with us a powerful, universal, and uplifting truth: that death is not the end of our story, nor does it sever the connection and love we feel with the most important people in our life."

—Kate Spencer, author of *The Dead Moms Club*

"Annie's provocative questions feel at once familiar and entirely fresh, and the kind of vulnerable storytelling that makes me want to hug her and, in fact, everyone. Annie's expertise as an ethnographer—as a professional empathy-generator—crackles on the page."

—Samara Bay, speech coach and author of *Permission to Speak*

ALWAYS
A
SIBLING

THE FORGOTTEN MOURNER'S GUIDE TO GRIEF

ALWAYS A SIBLING

ANNIE SKLAVER ORENSTEIN

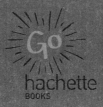

Go

hachette
BOOKS

New York

Hachette Go, an imprint of Hachette Books
Hachette Book Group
1290 Avenue of the Americas
New York, NY 10104
HachetteGo.com
Facebook.com/HachetteGo
Instagram.com/HachetteGo

First Edition: June 2024

Published by Hachette Go, an imprint of Hachette Book Group, Inc. The Hachette Go name and logo is a trademark of the Hachette Book Group.

The Hachette Speakers Bureau provides a wide range of authors for speaking events. To find out more, go to hachettespeakersbureau.com or email HachetteSpeakers@hbgusa.com.

Hachette Go books may be purchased in bulk for business, educational, or promotional use. For information, please contact your local bookseller or Hachette Book Group Special Markets Department at special.markets@hbgusa.com.

The publisher is not responsible for websites (or their content) that are not owned by the publisher.

Print book interior designed by Amy Quinn.

Library of Congress Cataloging-in-Publication Data

Names: Orenstein, Annie Sklaver, author.
Title: Always a sibling : the forgotten mourner's guide to grief / by Annie Sklaver Orenstein.
Description: New York, NY : Hachette Go, [2024] | Includes bibliographical references and index.
Identifiers: LCCN 2023054088 | ISBN 9780306831492 (hardcover) |
    ISBN 9780306831515 (ebook)
Subjects: LCSH: Siblings—Death. | Grief. | Bereavement—Psychological aspects.
Classification: LCC BF575.G7 O74 2024 | DDC 155.9/37—dc23/eng/20231221
LC record available at https://lccn.loc.gov/2023054088

ISBNs: 978-0-306-83149-2 (hardcover), 978-0-306-83151-5 (ebook)

Printed in the United States of America

LSC-C

Printing 1, 2024

To Sam. I love you, brother.

*In memory of Ben, Craig, Devra, Zach, Leah, Darrel, John, Megan, Greg,
and all the brothers and sisters who have left us too soon.*

Contents

Part II: Without

Part III: Within

Introduction

A FORGOTTEN MOURNER'S GUIDE TO GRIEF

I was a freshman in high school when my brother Ben, eight years older and light-years cooler than me, knocked on my door and announced we were going out to lunch. We picked up grinders and drove to the top of East Rock Park to set up our picnic. As I unwrapped my grinder, he began, "I know you're wondering why we're here."

Reader, I was not wondering; I thought maybe he just wanted to hang out with me, but okay. "I want you to be able to tell me things. High school is a really weird time, and sometimes it'll be great and other times it will be terrible. People say it's the best years of your life, but I don't think that's true. Or at least, I don't want it to be true. Why would you want your best years to be over by the time you turn eighteen and then you have to live another seventy years?"

The man had a point. He also had my rapt attention.

"So here's the deal. I want you to be open with me, but I realize it's hypocritical of me to expect you to tell me everything when you don't really know anything about my high school experience. You were so young when I was in high school, I didn't tell you anything. But now I'll tell you anything you want to know. I'm going to tell you all the stupid shit I did. And I hope you'll do the same with me."

1

My eyes grew wide. I was ten when he'd graduated high school, and those years had been a mystery to me. "You're going to tell me everything?" I said in disbelief.

"Everything," he responded. "Where should I start?"

The first story Ben told me was that the time he hurt his foot "at swim practice," he'd actually hurt it jumping off the low roof outside his bedroom window while sneaking out of the house.

"Why didn't you just walk out the back door?" I asked. I'd snuck out a few times already, and each time I'd simply walked out the sliding glass doors in our TV room.

"Annie. You can't just walk out the back door! It doesn't work like that."

"Sure it does. I did it last weekend. They don't turn on the alarm, and you can just pretend you're watching TV and then walk out once they're asleep."

He looked at me in shock. In that moment, for perhaps the first time in my life, I had the better answer. I had the smarter solution. I had taught him something. Goddamn, it felt good.

He started laughing his big, joyful laugh—the kind of laugh that could fill a stadium. He laughed harder and harder as he sputtered, "Oh my god I'm such an idiot. All those years, I could have just walked out the back door. I thought I was so good; I was so proud of myself. Annie, what else have you figured out? You're going to be so much better at this than I was."

In that moment our dynamic shifted. I wasn't the ten-year-old anymore. I wasn't him, I wasn't his peer, but I wasn't the baby either.

The afternoon wore on and he told me stories I'd never heard before. I was starting to get to know him as someone who made mistakes, some honest and some really stupid, but mistakes nonetheless. That day he was human.

I know that you have stories about your siblings too. Some that make you smile just to think about, others you fight back—trying to force them out of your mind as they get buried deeper and deeper. The relationship you shared with your sibling, no matter how fraught, had meaning and value. It has contributed to making you the person you are; it has brought you here to this moment.

Growing up I always gauged my worth and value, any redeeming qualities really, on my proximity to my older brothers. If I am Ben and Sam's sister, I can't be that bad because they are perfect. I didn't have to worry about who I was; I didn't need to have a distinct identity; I didn't have to *be* anything. I could just be their little sister, and for me that was enough. In the years since Ben's death, I struggled to find my way without his guidance. I had to be something on my own, but I did not *want* to be anything on my own. I went through the motions and managed to build a successful career as a researcher, conducting interviews and qualitative studies with people around the globe and translating my findings—their stories—into actionable business recommendations for my clients and employers. My studies have ranged from entertainment to terminal illness to social media, and my clients are some of the biggest companies in the world. And yet, I never felt that I was truly making a difference. I was gathering these incredibly powerful, life-altering stories from folks who might not otherwise have a voice, but then what? I felt the underlying need to use my superpower beyond the walls of a corporate office park and to share stories in a way that could help others who were struggling. And so, here we are. You and me. You and me and our brothers and sisters; here to share our stories in a way that will make a difference for the thousands of others who are grieving their siblings.

I ask questions for a living, questions that lead people to tell me their deepest secrets and silent regrets. The questions I ask open the doors for people to share the juicy stuff, the stuff they don't even admit to themselves.

I am so good at asking these questions, at eliciting the truth, that I never dared ask them of myself or my loved ones. I know the kinds of secrets people tell me, and I wasn't ready to explore my own version, my own story. Denial is my most favorite drug, especially when mixed with a healthy dose of self-loathing: chef's kiss. That is why I never understood self-help books.

You're telling me people want to turn inward and ask themselves these questions? What kind of self-inflicted torture nonsense is that? Turns out, when you ask the right questions, it isn't torture at all. These questions, the ones I ask myself, other grieving siblings, and you throughout this book, these are the questions that set us free.

If you picked up this book because you just lost a sibling, if the loss is fresh and you are still deeply in the shit (that's the technical term)—this book is still for you. But maybe the questions aren't, not yet. That's okay.

In the immediate aftermath of Ben's death, it felt like I was treading water in a toxic ocean. I knew that if my head went under, that would be it—I'd be a goner. I just needed to keep my head above water. That's it. But then there were the people standing on the shore, well-intentioned people, waving at me and calling out things like,

"HOW ARE YOUR PARENTS DOING?"

"EVERYTHING HAPPENS FOR A REASON!"

"WHO HAS BEN'S DOG?"

"CAN'T YOU SEE ME WAVING AT YOU? WHY AREN'T YOU WAVING BACK?"

Because if I wave at you, if I take even a moment's attention away from treading water, I will drown. Why can't anyone see that?

If you are still treading water, if you are simply trying to stay afloat, then that is what you need to focus on with all your might. The treading will get easier, and eventually you'll even be able to swim against the current. This book is your life jacket. It is your lighthouse. It is your rescue boat. And we will focus on getting you safely to shore.

Once you've warmed up and learned to breathe again, this book will help you put one foot in front of the other and begin to move through this strange new life.

And once you've regained your balance, this book will help you navigate your future with the love, legacy, and presence of your sibling.

When I was deep in the shit (again, technical term) it was hard to see the forest through the trees. Hell, I couldn't even see the trees through my tears. So I am going to lay it all out on the table here—no need for interpretation or guessing about what you will find on these pages. Plus, I am a researcher and I love tables.

WHAT THIS BOOK WILL GIVE YOU	WHAT THIS BOOK WILL NOT GIVE YOU
An opportunity to hear about the experiences of other grieving siblings in their own words	An idealized, rosy picture
Validation for your relationship and your loss	Your sibling back. I am so sorry.
A deep understanding that you are not alone in your grief	A quick fix
An excellent coaster	A time machine
Research-backed evidence on the types of grief and trauma unique to sibling loss, and the tools to address it	Answers to the questions of "why me?" and "why them?"
Exercises and activities designed and proven to help you process your grief	Homework
Tools and prompts to capture your sibling's legacy	Fear and isolation

Grief is like a choose your own adventure book. The worst choose your own adventure book ever written, and you can't even flip to the last page to cheat and then work your way backward. As the saying goes, the only way out is through—and we will get you through. This book will give you tools, ideas, inspiration, and community, but grief is not a checklist, and there will be twists and turns along the way. One of the hardest parts of grief, for me, was the realization that I needed to be an active participant in my own healing. All I wanted to do was fall asleep and wake up to learn it was all a dream. I didn't want to *work* to feel better, I wanted my brother to hug me and help me feel better. That's how it had always been. I didn't know—nor did I want to learn—how to survive on my own.

The tools in this book will help you be that active participant and put you in control of how you proceed. How will we do that? By creating your own Mourner's User Manual (MUM). *You might roll your eyes but please don't write me off quite yet—hear me out.* Through the activities in this book, you'll create a resource that you can refer back to when critical thought and social skills leave you (which they often do when grieving). It will take the guesswork out of what you need and how you'll get it. Most of the MUM-specific activities begin in Part II: Without, as we grapple with the reality of our loss. For that reason, you may want to read chapters out of order, focusing on the one most relevant to your current state.

You might want to come back and reread sections later.

You might not be ready for the exercises, and that's okay, you can always come back to them. There's no right or wrong way to grieve, that's why it's so hard.

This book isn't going anywhere. It will be here for you whenever you're ready for it—maybe that's today, maybe that's in ten years. Grieving a sibling can be a torturously lonely endeavor, but you are not alone. Your grief is not forgotten. Not here. Not with me, and not with the other people reading along with you.

We can remember them.

We can honor them.

We can honor our relationships.

We can learn to feel their presence.

The most important piece of our journey will be words. The words of other grieving siblings who have lent themselves to this book, and your words. Yes, yours.

Words can be a very scary thing. They can include truths that we are not yet ready to face, but words do not need to be feared. They do not need to own you. You can use as many words as you want to answer the activities in this book, and no one will ever need to read them. Hell, you don't even need to reread them. The greatest value is in the experience of writing them down in the first place, by hand if possible, as the act of writing itself is shown to increase brain activity associated with memory, imaginary visualization, and recall. If you are brave enough to write these words on the page, they will help you remember.

In *On Grief and Grieving*, Elisabeth Kübler-Ross and David Kessler write, "Tell your tale, because it reinforces that your loss mattered." They continue, explaining that storytelling "helps dissipate the pain . . . telling your story often and in detail is primal for the grieving process."[1] Dozens of grieving siblings have generously shared their stories with us in this book, folks who have lost siblings to drugs, mental illness, physical illness, accidents, and violence, some best friends, some estranged. I need you to know, before you even begin this book, that your stories matter. All of your stories matter.

Throughout this book you will be guided through therapeutic exercises that support narrative reconstruction, a practice involving the detailed written reconstruction of memories and what those memories mean to us, which is proven to be effective in reducing the symptoms of depression and complicated grief.

The stories that dissipate the pain are the ones that acknowledge and address it—they are the stories with emotion. In *Rising Strong*, author and researcher Brené Brown discusses the importance of recognizing and getting curious about our emotions in a process she calls Reckoning with Emotion. This is not a process that feels good or comes naturally, but sometimes it's the hardest things that help us the most. Due to the intense, surprising, and dark feelings grief evokes within us, coupled with society's inability to accept that grief is something to live with—not get over—Brown has found that grief is the emotion we fear the most.[2]

Embarking on this work is scary, but it's not as scary as what you've already been through. If you're here, holding this book, then you're ready. You are stronger than you think, and you can do this—at your own pace and in your own time, you can do this.

My brother always loved song lyrics. He believed them to be the highest form of poetry. His diaries are full of lyrics—in some places he transcribed full songs, while in others simply a word or two. Now that he's gone, I feel his presence most when I'm listening to music. Certain songs will remind me of him, even songs he'd never heard. Others give me that warm feeling like he's sending through a message from whatever magical land he currently inhabits.

One such song is "For a Dancer," written by Jackson Browne upon learning of the death of a friend, with its haunting brilliance that speaks to the pain of death and the joy of life. A soldier my brother deployed with said that one afternoon on base he was listening to Jackson Browne and Ben walked through a cloud of dust, dancing and singing along with this song. "He was singing about death," the soldier told me, "with this big ol' grin across his face." If you can, find a quiet place at a quiet moment, and listen to that song. I recommend using headphones so the words really envelop you. These will be our instructions as we look toward tomorrow; we will keep a fire burning in our eyes and pay attention to the open sky. You never know what will be coming down.

Music will guide us throughout this book. At one point I'll even ask you to create a playlist of your own. There will be moments when I use song lyrics to express the emotions that I have no other words for, or to convey universal truths too poetic to top. While each of our losses is unique, and the loss of a sibling is unique beyond that, there are others who understand. To hear them in your ears and your mind can help you feel less alone, and I invite you to seek out those voices whenever you can.

You will also not be alone because you will have me. You and me, we're climbing to the top of East Rock, and I'm going to tell you all the dumb stuff I did. Not because I don't expect you to do plenty of your own dumb stuff, you will do plenty, but at least you'll know you're not the only one. My greatest wish is that you begin to tell your stories too, because yours is a story that needs to be told. We might not ever be whole again, but together we can fill that void with love and meaning.

In Ben's many diaries he revisits the idea of writing a book, and of what that book might be.

In one passage, he describes his book as

Something that clarifies the world around us, or opens new questions, new ways of seeing or understanding experiences. Something that encourages you when you are struggling, comforts when you are overwhelmed, makes you smile when you are cold, reassures you that you are not the first, nor the only person to go through this hectic, crazy, funny, scary, cold, loud world. Like a hot, sugary mug of tea when you hike too late into a dark campsite, covered in sweat, cold and scared and relieved that you will make it to a safe bed tonight. That hot sugary mug should be this book.

Ben isn't here to write his book, and that's even more of a reason why I need that hot, sugary mug. If you're reading this, then you need it too. That's what we will do here together. Using research, storytelling, and a pinch of creativity, we will explore new questions and ways of understanding our experiences, we will find comfort and reassurance, and we will take the first steps in the new world without our siblings by our side. It doesn't matter if you lost your sibling yesterday, twenty years ago, or if they were lost before you were even born—this book is for you. These chapters, and their activities, are designed to meet you exactly where you are so that we can walk forward together.

A Note on Sources

One day, during the writing of this book, I was meeting with a senior executive at the tech company I work for, and he asked what the topic of my book was. After fumbling through my response, he asked if I had experienced the loss of a sibling. In a moment of true unprofessionalism, I guffawed and exclaimed, "Oh my god can you imagine if I hadn't!?" For a split second I *did* consider answering, "Nah, I'm an only child" just to mess with him, but I stopped myself. Truth is, it's not a bad question! I knew why he was asking—I'm a researcher and, as such, my job is to synthesize and distill the experiences of others without injecting my own biases into my findings. That's what he's used to seeing from me. This book is not that, at least not exactly. This book, and the stories it contains, belongs to the hundreds of people who so graciously participated in my research; and it belongs to me (biases and all).

In addition to the many academic studies and grief texts cited in these pages, much of this book is based on my own primary research. The first phase of research consisted of a survey that was completed by 350 grieving siblings between late March and early May 2022. The survey responses were then evaluated across different dimensions, including birth order, relationship health, cause of death, age at the time of death, and length of time since the death occurred. The siblings who took the time to complete the survey included painful details and thoughtful reflections, and this book would not be possible without them.

I then conducted forty in-depth interviews with grieving siblings across the dimensions previously mentioned. Each of these interviews lasted anywhere from one to three hours and illuminated sibling grief in ways I hadn't previously considered. In interview after interview, I was stunned by the honesty, vulnerability, and dedication shown by each participant. Many told me that they were doing it for you, dear reader, so that you might feel a little less alone. Some names have been changed at the request of the participant. This book would not be possible without them.

Part I

With

one

The Day

I don't know what happens when people die / can't seem to grasp it as hard as I try / it's like a song I can hear playing right in my ear / but I can't sing, I can't help listening.

—Jackson Browne

Every grieving sibling has a death day. The day the world opened up and swallowed our past, present, and future in one gulp. In studies on sibling loss, researchers note that all respondents—no matter how many years have passed since the death of their sibling—cannot recount The Day without showing physical signs of distress.[1] In my own research I have seen the same. I've interviewed people who have lost their sibling within the past year, and others whose loss was decades earlier; I have yet to speak with a single person who can tell the story without watery eyes, a sniffling nose, tear-streaked cheeks, or a tremble in their voice. As one grieving sibling explained, "It's been twenty-seven years and one day and I can still smell the air the morning my sister died and I found her."

It's hard to know where to begin when explaining to someone what happened on The Day. How can you fully understand what happened without the backstory? What got us here, to this terrible, terrible place. How can someone possibly understand what we lost without first understanding what we had?

I'll start my story with the day Anna Lifshitz bought the house at 16 East Walk in the spring of 1942 (don't worry, I'll skip a lot of decades in between). Her options were limited since Beach Park, the small shoreline community where the house was located, was the only one in Connecticut that would allow Jews to own property. That same year Anna's son-in-law, Dr. Joe Sklaver, deployed to the Horn of Africa as a military doctor during WWII. Both Joe and Anna were living lives vastly different from their Jewish relatives in Germany, and each was doing their best to make a better life for their family during a terrifyingly uncertain time. They were brought together by Anna's daughter, Vi, who had married Joe two years earlier and was now pregnant with their first son, a boy named Neal whom Joe would not meet until he was three years old. Anna bought the house as (what I assume to be) a distraction from the realities of their life, but I'll never really know her motivations. Perhaps she just craved the peaceful sound of waves breaking on the beach. Or perhaps, if you believe in things like fate and purpose, 1942 was the year when both Anna and Joe set into motion the events that would define their family for generations to come.

Sixty years after Anna purchased that home at 16 East Walk, it remained the cornerstone of her family and legacy, but Vi and Joe had become too old to care for the little cottage. I can only tell you that because they're both dead now. If Vi were alive, I wouldn't dare call her "old" in print, even if she were in her nineties. That woman would have eaten me alive; dentures be damned.

My father, the third of their four boys, was the only one left in Connecticut, so it made sense that he and my mother take over the cottage. While my parents made it their own in some respects, it remained the central hub for all my aunts, uncles, and dozens of cousins. The house itself had become the family's matriarch, and Beach Park was everyone's safe place. How privileged we were to have had a place so sacred that it blocked out the world for decades.

On the afternoon of October 2, 2009, my mom was in the Beach Park bubble waiting for my dad to get home from work and preparing to go out for dinner with some friends.

Five o'clock came and went without a word. She wavered between concern and annoyance—where was he and why wasn't he answering his phone?

On his way to the cottage, Dad had stopped at their home to pick up the mail and open some windows. It would be stuffy there, having been empty for the past five months. That was all he intended to do. Pick up the mail and open the windows. Shortly after he walked in, there was a knock at the door, and he saw what every military family dreads: two soldiers in uniform, sent to tell an unsuspecting parent that their child had been killed. I wonder about those soldiers sometimes. How many times have they seen a person's entire life and dreams of the future crumble before their eyes as they deliver devastating news that will change these families forever?

Somehow, Dad drove himself to that cottage where he'd grown up, the cottage that housed some of the best memories our family had formed over generations. He drove slowly, hands on ten and two, as the soldiers followed behind him. Mom, no longer pretending to be calm, called him every ten minutes to see where he was and what was taking so long—it wasn't like him to be this late. He didn't answer, he just drove. Thirty minutes later he pulled into the driveway and stepped out of the car, pale and trembling as he faced his wife.

"Ben was killed today in Afghanistan," he said in a calm, level voice. She must have heard him wrong. That wasn't possible.

"Ben was killed today in Afghanistan," he repeated.

"Ben was killed today in Afghanistan," as he walked toward her.

"Ben was killed today in Afghanistan," over and over, as if he had been rehearsing as he drove. He had.

Then she saw them, the soldiers walking up the driveway behind him.

From the doorway of the cottage, my mother stumbled backward into the kitchen and crumpled to the floor.

The soldiers walked through the door and immediately sat beside her on the floor, one on each side, as they recounted that day's events just as they had for my father. They calmly, patiently, and empathically tore our world apart while sitting on the floor of the kitchen that Anna had established as a safe haven to avoid the horrors of war seventy years earlier.

My brother Sam and I remained blissfully unaware for only a few minutes longer than our parents. Sam and his wife, Wendi, were on a rare date night as I babysat their one-year-old son. The baby was asleep and I was enjoying their premium cable subscription, waiting for my dinner delivery to arrive, when the door opened and Sam and Wendi stumbled in. Startled, I walked toward the door to ask why they were home so soon, and they surrounded me, sandwiching me in a hug, as Sam whispered, "It's Ben."

"But he's okay," I said. I didn't ask; I didn't think it was a question.

"No," he replied.

"Annie, Ben's gone."

I don't know how I got back to the couch, but I remember sitting there, rocking back and forth, repeating "this wasn't supposed to happen" over and over and over. The truth is, I *did* think this was going to happen. I'd been convinced of it. Our family was too perfect; we had it too good. Our parents remained happily married as my friends' parents divorced; we siblings got along great while others struggled with estrangement and betrayal. Nothing bad ever happened to us, and I knew enough to know that that isn't realistic—that isn't life. I'd spent my entire life waiting for our bad thing to happen—the tragedy that would define our family. That was why I'd been so terrified for Ben to deploy; I was convinced he wouldn't return. I'm not psychic. I believe in psychics, but I am not clairvoyant; I am a very neurotic Jew with a diagnosed anxiety disorder, and my brother was deployed to an active war zone. But then it happened, and suddenly I was convinced that I'd been wrong all along—this was *not* supposed to happen. This was not the way our story was going to end. Ben, Sam, and I would grow old together—that was the way it was supposed to be.

Sam and I stood on his back porch smoking cigarettes and hugging, only removing an arm when we needed to take another drag. Sam told me that there were soldiers waiting at our parents' house with the news. After they'd shared the news with him, Sam told them that I was sitting in his apartment, that he would tell me, and he did.

Sam had to tell his baby sister that their big brother was dead.

He was the only big brother now. Thrust into a new family dynamic that none of us wanted.

I witnessed over thirty-five siblings recount their Death Day. With my heart in my throat and a box of tissues by my side, I heard stories of people who found their siblings incapacitated by suicide, watched as they were ravaged by disease, navigated the trauma of a sudden violent death, and wrestled with conflicting emotions upon hearing that their estranged sibling had died. Stories of addiction, mental illness, homicide, suicide, accidents, and disease—across an incalculable combination of relationship types, traumas, shared histories, and external forces. I want to share a few of those stories with you now because my story might look nothing like your own. Perhaps none of these do, but I hope you can find a single emotion that reflects your own. A kernel of experience that helps you feel less alone and may even inspire you to put your own story into words.

Jessica was the oldest of three sisters. They were all adopted, but Jessica was quick to explain to me that while she and her middle sister were adopted as infants, their younger sister had been six, the child of two addicts, and love could not heal her wounds. Mae started using drugs when she was twelve and spent her twenties and early thirties in and out of prison.

"It was better, actually, when she was in prison," Jessica explained to me. "When she was in jail at least we knew where she was, we knew that she's okay. Even if she's still using, the grade of drugs they're getting is so low you actually feel safe."

Three years ago, shortly after Mae had been released from prison, Jessica got a call from her mother while she was driving home with her two young children. "I have to tell you something," her mom started before announcing, "Mae's dead."

Jessica pulled to the side of the road unable to breathe. She'd always known overdose was possible, perhaps even probable, but she'd also held out hope that her sister would be "the one that beats it." Jessica got out of the car and doubled over on the side of the road in tears, her five-year-old asking what was happening out the window.

"My sister died. Mama's sister died. Mae's dead. My sister dead," Jessica repeated as she struggled to breathe again.

They didn't know her. Her children had never met her sister.

Stephanie is the youngest of ten children and the only girl. She has nine older brothers, her "tiny little patriarchy," she calls it. She had a special bond with her brother Andy, fifteen years her senior. When she told me about him, she said that it was a "privilege" to even be able to talk about him, he was just that special. Andy tested HIV positive in 1987, early in the AIDS epidemic. Their parents were both medical professionals, and Andy's illness was never a secret within the family.

> My dad is a doctor. My mom is a nurse. The way that they coped with disease, or death, or diagnoses, was to just get practical, boots on the ground, medical. Asking all the doctors "have you checked this, have you done this, have you done that," and I remember Andy wishing Papa would stop trying to be his doctor and just try to be his dad. And it wasn't just my parents. Three of our brothers were doctors too, and I remember these talks where they'd try to come up with new things to try, new ways to treat the virus.

In 1991, when Stephanie was fifteen years old, Andy took a turn for the worse and was hospitalized on and off for months. She'd become very used to hearing her dad on the phone with other doctors and patients (not just Andy), discussing medical issues in the middle of the living room for all to hear. This call had started normally enough, with her father asking for stats and vitals, but then the conversation changed. This was not a normal medical call.

My brother had gone into cardiac arrest. They had been performing CPR for fifteen minutes, and they told my dad it wasn't working, but he advised them to go for another fifteen minutes. He told them they had to keep going. That's when my mom got on the phone and quietly said, "You've got to let him go, Dick. You've got to let him go." Hearing them . . . hearing that call. My dad was saying, "You've got to keep doing this. You've got to." He was just trying to be the doctor in the room, saying, "No, do this. Try this. Have you tried this? Have you tried this?" And my mom as a nurse going, "It's happened." My father finally said, "Okay, we've got to let him go" and began to cry. To watch him give up like that, even though it was already too late by the time they called . . . It was thirty years ago, and I can't think of that moment without crying.

Hugo and his younger sister were best friends. Entering their forties, they still spoke every day in one way or another. Then there was the day his sister didn't show up to work, and he found her in her apartment.

There are so many stories. And many of us all thought that Day was the worst of it, that nothing could be worse than that moment, those words—but we were wrong. I know now that it gets worse before it gets better, but that night, my night, I didn't think "worse" was even a possibility.

In Chapter 14 we're going to focus on telling your story, on owning the narrative that is your life and loss—however complicated that may be—but we need to go slow. For those who have experienced a traumatic loss or are experiencing PTSD or traumatic grief, remembering the day can be extremely triggering and reactivate your grief. It's essential that you take care of yourself above all else. Throughout this book, and beyond it, remember that you come first. Take breaks when needed and don't do anything that feels too overwhelming.

If you are experiencing trauma, it's a good idea to work with a therapist who can support your healing. If you don't have a therapist yet, visit PsychologyToday.com and on the top of the page you'll see "find a therapist." Look for someone in your area who specializes in grief and trauma.

two

The Sibling Relationship

I hate my sister, she's such a bitch. / She acts as if she doesn't even know that I exist. / But I would do anything to let her know I care. / But I am only talking to myself 'cause she isn't there.

—Juliana Hatfield

While conducting research for this book I uncovered plenty of facts and statistics that piqued my interest, many that confirmed or disproved an implicit hunch I'd had; and then there were the few that truly stopped me in my tracks and reframed everything. One of those moments came while reading the work of sibling and family expert Dr. Susan McHale, who noted that more children grow up in households with siblings than with fathers.

More children share a home, a roof, a life, with siblings than with fathers.

When I spoke with Dr. McHale, she explained that siblings share an understanding of the interior of the family, and as a result, no one knows you in the same way a sibling does. That sibling insight—the understanding of not just who you are but why you are—is a theme we will continue to revisit throughout the book. In this chapter, we will wrestle with exactly how influential the sibling relationship is—for better or worse.

In childhood, siblings (on average) spend more time together than with anyone else, including their parents.[1] In *The Sibling Effect*, author Jeff Kluger shares how the psychiatrist Daniel Shaw described, "Parents serve the same big-picture role as doctors on grand rounds. Siblings are like the nurses on the ward; they're there every day."[2] Biologically and in general, it should be our longest shared relationship, extending beyond the death of a parent and beginning before any kind of adult partnership is formed. Research into identity development has shown that siblings are critical to forming one's own distinct personality. They are our "touchstones" and references on the road to personal identity.[3] This doesn't mean we form our identities to be similar to our siblings; often it's quite the opposite. Sibling de-identification is a means of avoiding the pitfalls of sibling rivalry by intentionally trying to be different from each other.

As the youngest of three, I actively sought my place in the world in reference to my brothers. Ben was the smart one, the straight-A student-athlete who could do no wrong, and Sam was the funny one who could charm even our meanest grandma and always (always, always) make me laugh. I was . . . the girl? The one with good hair? Certainly not as smart as Ben (in my opinion) or as funny as Sam (in anyone's opinion), I had no natural aptitude for sports, and while I had creative ideas, my fine art skills were . . . lacking. In my mind, there was no use trying to be the smart one if I wasn't going to be the smartest, no use trying to be the charismatic or popular one when I was already the victim of middle school bullies. Without knowing such a phenomenon existed, I spent years grappling with sibling de-identification without ever truly finding my place. I didn't hold resentment toward my brothers, who had essentially "called dibs" on their identities by simply getting here first, but it's not difficult to see how that kind of resentment could grow and thrive in a competitive or unhealthy way. In hindsight, I know that my family had plenty of space for me to be smart, funny, or a combination of just about anything; but thirteen-year-old Annie didn't see it that way.

Perhaps because we all carved our own distinct identities, or because of our age difference, or because of pure luck, my brothers were my most treasured best friends. Other grieving siblings I spoke with carried similar sentiments, often describing their sibling as their "first best friend," "true life partner," and "the most influential person in my life."

"We were the only people we had to survive," Breanne explained. "There are no memories he wasn't part of, and we were happiest when we were together." Chris described his siblings as "odd safety nets. Given the right one you can trust them with anything. Life ends up scarier without them."

Life ends up scarier without them.

In *The Sibling Effect*, Jeff Kluger writes of his own siblings: "The four of us, we came to know at a very deep level, were a unit—a loud, messy, brawling, loyal, loving, lasting unit. We felt much, much stronger that way than we did as individuals. And whenever the need arose, we knew we'd be able to call on that strength."[4]

Like all relationships, sibling relationships fall on a spectrum. My relationship with my brothers falls in the "you three get along so well it's kind of creepy" end of the spectrum. But for some, especially those whose siblings struggled physically or mentally during their life, their relationships might not look "typical" from the outside—even still there is a bond between them that is deeper than the circumstances of their relationship.

Speaking to mourners who had these close positive connections with their siblings illuminated moments of small, simple pleasures and rituals. Kenny and Sarah both told me they called their siblings every day when they'd get in the car. Kenny described their routine, grinning: "We'd call each other on our way to work every day. We drove opposite directions on the interstate, and when we passed each other he'd always flip me off."

How is it that getting the middle finger from your sibling can be such a universal sign of affection? When I was in sixth grade, my brother Sam and I were in a car accident, and as we were lying in that hospital room next to each other, I'd turn every few minutes to make sure Sam was okay (he was), and each time we made eye contact he'd give me the finger—that's how I knew he was okay—we were okay. For me, that was the perfect encapsulation of unique sibling love.

RELATIONSHIP FACTORS

Studies have shown that the quality of the sibling relationship is linked to psychological and subjective well-being throughout our life span, and it is essential to acknowledge—and explore—the truth that the quality of this relationship isn't always very good.[5] We need to make space for relationships that were imperfect, strained, abusive, estranged, or otherwise fraught. Those relationships still need to be mourned. Just because you didn't have a positive relationship doesn't mean you won't grieve.

Dr. McHale didn't sugarcoat the all-too-common negative realities of these relationships. In her work, she's found that the number one area of disagreement between a parent and child centers on how that child gets along with their siblings. It's not about how often the siblings themselves fight, but rather how often the parents have a conflict with their child as a result of their relationship with a sibling.

The reality of conflict within the sibling relationship often isn't much better. A 1980s study found that 82 percent of siblings engaged in some form of physical violence against another sibling, and nearly half had hit a sibling with some kind of object.[6] According to McHale, not much has changed since. As she told me when we spoke,

> People who've looked at family conflict have found that there's, on average, more physical aggression and violence between siblings than domestic violence between partners or parents, or child abuse. But because the sibling relationship isn't that important, parents, at least in Western cultures, don't take it as seriously. You can have a sibling who's a bully, a sibling who

is abusive behind the parents' back, and their response is "that's just the way kids are."

I tell this story sometimes when I give a talk on siblings, told to me by one of my colleagues. He was watching his kids' swim team warm up before a race, and this boy jumps into the pool and starts dunking a girl under the water. She's gasping and trying to get away and the lifeguard runs over. The boy says something to the lifeguard, and the lifeguard shrugs and walks away, leaving the kid to continue dunking this younger little girl. And what did he say?

"It's only my sister."

One of the first questions I asked Dr. McHale was why there has been so little research done on siblings beyond her own (extensive) work. She explained that it is a difficult relationship to study because there are so many variables to account for: sex and gender, birth order, single-parent versus dual-parent households, number of siblings, socioeconomic status, and the list goes on and on. In this chapter and beyond, I'll be explicit about the factors I believe significantly impact the quality of sibling relationships. First up . . .

BIRTH ORDER

Younger Sibling: Many of the younger siblings I spoke with viewed the older as a guidepost—a preview of their own future and a parental figure all in one. And while olders were idolized, that doesn't mean they lived up to, or embraced, their elevated status. In a survey of over 350 bereaved siblings, respondents used words like "protector," "invincible," and "caregiver" to describe their older siblings. But, and I cannot stress this enough, it does not mean their older siblings actually were perfect. As one respondent put it, "He loved being a big brother, even though he wasn't particularly good at it."

I'll be honest—Ben and Sam were/are particularly good at it. I took my first steps to Ben, simply because he called my name. I saw that same love and devotion in Devin's eyes when he talked about his big brother:

My first memory is hearing his voice. I was in a crib in New York City and I heard his voice, this is me on the grid now—shocked onto the grid for the first time—and it was his voice saying, 'Can I go wake Devin?' He would take care of me. He was always like that with me.

Anne-Lyse described her older sister as a second mother, but as a child "I didn't understand why she wanted to play mom." Julie's parents were gone a lot so her older sister took on the caregiver role, cooking them dinner and ensuring homework was complete. She thought they were so special because they never fought—and they were. Julie told me that as a child she'd listen to "Wind Beneath My Wings" on cassette and think the song was written about them.

The perception that the older sibling knows best and guides the way certainly gets more complicated as we age, but it doesn't really go away. Those big brothers and sisters who cared for us so deeply, though sometimes in their own flawed ways, often saw things in us that we struggled to see in ourselves. As Anne-Lyse put it, "My sister thought that I was whoever I wanted to become."

Older Sibling: Speaking with older siblings (as the youngest myself), I was surprised how often their perspective complemented that of the younger siblings. Many do see themselves as a parent figure, responsible for the current and future well-being of the younger. Sarah, the middle of three, desperately wanted a baby before her brother was born. Once he was finally here, she saw him as *her* baby. When he was in kindergarten, he got on the wrong school bus and Sarah blamed herself—she should have looked out for him. As they got older, Sarah watched him veer off track again and again, first in fifth grade when he was caught smoking cigarettes. Her parents told her not to worry, that this wasn't her problem, but it was *her baby*, and as someone much closer to the realities of youth culture, she could see what was coming.

Many, like Sarah, were aware that their parents didn't want them involved in the parenting of their younger siblings (remember those conflicts?), but they couldn't stop. When Rheanna's parents tried to sleep train her baby brother, she would sneak into his room and rock him to sleep: "I wanted to be the parent I never had. I wanted to be the parent he needed. I wanted him to feel heard."

I knew I idolized my big brothers—*everyone* knew I idolized my big brothers—but I never understood the older sibling's perspective until I first read Ben's diaries a decade after his death.

> Sam and I went for a walk so I got to talk to the boy, something about brothers. Just the word—there's a bond, something shared. I look up to him and he looks up to me. I'm sure Sam and I will be close forever. Annie and I have a different relationship—pure love. We could go out and have a great time together. We do. But it's different. We love each other not out of admiration but because she's my sister and I'm her brother. That's all, that's how it is.

The way he uses "boy" to describe his younger brother who, at sixteen, stood about six foot three inches tall is just perfect. My Grandpa Joe lived to be an incredible ninety-seven years old. He'd lost one sister decades earlier (my namesake), but he still had his baby sister, Evelyn. I'm not sure I ever actually heard him call her "Evelyn"; in all my memories he referred to her only as "my baby sister." Evelyn is 103 years old now, and I have no doubt that if my grandfather were alive, he'd still be calling her his baby sister.

PHYSICAL ILLNESS

When physical illness is present in the sibling relationship, it can often hang in the air as a weight whose shape and details cannot be defined. For siblings who experienced disability or illness from birth, it was all they ever knew. Of his older sister, one brother told me, "I only ever knew her as someone who could not speak, could not walk, and could really only communicate with a smile or by crying. I loved her very much and it was all I ever knew."

When the illness presents in childhood, many siblings told me that, in hindsight, they knew little of the reality surrounding the diagnosis.

Julie's sister, who cared for her so deeply, was diagnosed with lupus when Julie was only twelve. While she could tell something was wrong, she had no details to define it and was kept mostly in the dark. In adulthood her family often didn't tell her of her sister's hospitalizations until after the fact. "You feel guilty for living life while they're sick," she told me. "My sister would say, 'I might not live that long,' but I couldn't comprehend that. I realize now she was more open with her own kids than with me." To comprehend her sister's mortality would be to comprehend her own, because as our longest relationship, we expect to die at the same time as our siblings. It's why so many report that they assume they, too, will die shortly after losing a sibling (we'll discuss this mortality wake-up call more in Chapter 10).

For siblings struggling with physical illness as adults, some begin processing the reality and spring to action, while others remain in denial. When Devin's brother was hospitalized for ulcerative colitis as an adult, "it presented me with the scale of love I have for this human being." He would sit beside his brother's hospital bed and hold his hand every night from 8:00 p.m. to 6:00 a.m., "pretending everything was okay."

Sarah's big sister was terrified of falling asleep when she was hospitalized, so Sarah would sit by her bedside and hold her hand each night as she fell asleep. Julie would paint her sister's toenails bright colors. Of all the themes, patterns, and threads I unraveled in my research, holding hands in the hospital was one of the most beautiful and heart-wrenching of all.

TRAUMA

The type of closeness shared by siblings can't be replicated because of the shared childhood—and shared trauma—that formed us as individuals and as a unit. While I heard many beautiful stories of the sibling relationship, they were by no means perfect or without their fair share (or perhaps unfair share) of trauma—both from within the sibling relationship and in the environment surrounding it. One clear pattern that emerged from my research was that external trauma seemed to bond siblings together while internal trauma drove them apart. This could be a form of compensatory process that we know exists, but researchers haven't yet determined the point at which the compensation is triggered. This could also be seen as evidence to support attachment theory, which states that it is in our biology to seek closeness in times of need. We are wired to find a guardian or attachment figure with whom we can foster stable emotional bonds in times of need, who can provide a positive model of self. When that time of need is caused by a parent or guardian (intentionally or not), siblings naturally turn to each other as their attachment figure. As one sibling put it, "We were raised by a narcissistic mother, and we were trying to navigate the lack of love and acceptance with only each other as children. We endured a lot of trauma in our lives, but we always had one another." This bond is their attempt to protect themselves from the adjustment problems that can come with negative family dynamics.[7] At some point, it's not one sibling against the other; it's The Siblings against the world.

It's you and me against the world.

Then there are other times when the conflict, and the trauma, emerges from within the sibling relationship. In those situations, when one is abusive toward their sibling(s) and immediate family members, that trauma tears us apart. At a young age, Laura's interactions with her older brother were much like what Dr. McHale described: they would play fight, and since she was so much younger and smaller, she had a speed advantage. But then she paused: "We would, like, play fight a lot, but maybe it was a real fight? Looking back, I can tell that he was obviously using full force on this little girl. He was so big, and he definitely accidentally hurt me a lot of the time." She visibly shakes the question out of her mind and continues, "We just had a very standard, close sibling relationship."

[[record scratch]]

Why is this normalized? Why is it considered a normal close sibling relationship when one uses full physical force on the other? It may come as no surprise that Laura's physical safety continued to be thrown into question for the entirety of her older brother's life. When she was fourteen she was in his room looking for video games and instead found used syringes. Her mother had already told her that he'd been using heroin, and when he moved back home under the condition that he stopped using, Laura told her mother what she'd found. Laura was not protected. When her mother confronted him about the syringes, she told him that Laura had been the one to find them, and that was when he turned.

> It was one of the biggest fights in our relationship and he threatened violence. I remember his eyes, they looked completely sad and black. My mom had to get in between us physically and it was just really, really scary. I'd never seen them like that before. Even though I'd been on the receiving end of a lot of more, like, lighthearted physical threats and some more serious ones, but it never felt like I was actually in danger. This time I knew I was in danger.

Laura ran from her house, at fourteen, and stayed with a friend. She called her mother that night and gave her the ultimatum: "It's either me or him in the house. And she didn't make a decision, so that kind of meant the default—she chose him. So I went to live with my dad for a while." By the time he died, Laura had already grieved their relationship many times over.

This pattern of moving in and out of their lives, bouncing between safety and fear, was seen in many relationships in which one sibling struggled with addiction and/or mental health issues.

MENTAL ILLNESS

Depending on when their sibling's struggle with mental illness began, and their role in the family unit, surviving siblings I spoke with had a wide range of insight into their sibling's reality and perhaps the highest number of unanswered questions.

When Rob described his youngest sister's struggle with mental health as a teen, he explained, "My parents did a lot in terms of shielding the other kids from what was really going on, and the reality is, part of her struggle became just what it was like to live in our house. Looking back there was a lack of appreciation for what was really going on because it's really hard to understand mental illness when you're a teenager."

Molly and Kim (who have never met) both experienced childhood with brothers who struggled with mental illness, and both were kept in the dark. After Molly's brother was put on lithium at age eleven, he went into foster care while she remained with their parents. She would visit her brother in foster care, but those visits were confusing and sporadic. "He was never allowed to think he was anything except a bad kid," she confided, "except when he was with me." Decades later, she still doesn't know why or how their parents made that decision.

Kim's story is all too similar. When she was in eighth grade, her brother was sent away to a therapeutic boarding school. "I didn't know what he'd done to be sent away. We have knives in the kitchen, so I didn't understand why he couldn't have scissors in his room." Along with confusion came the resentment that so often accompanies sibling relationships. Resentment that he couldn't just "get his shit together and be the older brother." Kim was only permitted to visit her brother once a year during this time, but she was quick to assure me that she'd written regularly. "Every Thursday I wrote him; I added reminders in my school planner. Every Thursday." That small detail, the image of that reminder beside homework assignments and middle school notes, made me cry.

ADDICTION

I've struggled with whether to group addiction and mental health together because many people believe addiction is, itself, a type of mental illness. And so many of the stories of mental health struggles in adolescents progressed to addiction, but some did not. For that reason, I'll often address addiction on its own.

It was Sara, one of those older sisters who referred to her brother as "my baby," who described the impact of addiction so succinctly: "It is hell on earth to love someone so much and watch them struggle so deeply." Her empathy for him made it evident why she pursued a career as a school psychiatrist. "He was my baby and I'd rather him die than spend life in prison. He must have been in so much pain." Through tears, she told me, "I love him so much that I couldn't imagine him living like that any longer."

One of the elements of addiction that stood out to me was the complex combination of guilt and relief that followed the death of their siblings. This is not to say they did not mourn—they did. They'd been mourning for much of their sibling's life, long before their death. Many told me they felt they'd lost their siblings years before when they lost the person they once were.

Juliet's brother's addiction impacted their entire family on an individual and group level. She explained that his addiction "took over" their family, and she and her other siblings couldn't truly celebrate their successes. Those siblings who were doing well ended up ignored because they didn't need the lifesaving interventions their brother so desperately required. As a result, Juliet's loss was accompanied by a sense of relief. "It was pure relief, and I didn't feel guilty about it. It had been thirty-five years. He can no longer create issues."

When Caity told me about her older brother, she described their relationship as being "each other's diaries." She wanted to keep his secrets, and he always made it clear that he didn't want her to feel his pain. But it was as if, from childhood, she knew she'd lose him. She was shielded from the reality of his first rehab stay when she was in fourth grade, but she always just knew. "In every photo of us," she stressed, "I am physically holding onto him." Now, I come from a family of huggers, so I didn't comprehend the gravity of her statement until she pulled out a family photo in which she is tightly clinging to his arm—not in an annoying-little-sister way, but like someone desperately trying to keep him from floating away.

ESTRANGEMENT OR INDIFFERENCE

In my survey of grieving siblings, I asked respondents to describe their relationship with their deceased sibling. Many of those responses described not love or hate—but indifference. The relationship of two people who have nothing in common except their parentage. These responses, at least on paper, appeared almost startlingly casual:

"We weren't particularly close. I couldn't tell you who his friends were. We used to just coexist."

"It felt like he lived a completely separate life I wasn't part of."

"We were always really different. I'd never be friends with her if she wasn't my sibling."

"We didn't fight; we were just different people."

Upon further investigation, it became clear that the lack of a relationship was mutual in some cases, and in others one sibling had cut ties with the other. I'll refer to these instances of intentionally severing the relationship by one party as estrangement. It's different from the indifference described above, as many who've experienced indifference still had that sibling floating around—appearing at family functions and being civil over the dinner table. When the connection had been severed intentionally, however, the impact was significantly different. Estrangement triggers its own type of grief, mourning the relationship that existed and the broken family unit. But estrangement grief isn't the same as death grief because estrangement isn't *always* permanent, and some hold on to a thread of hope for reconciliation. That hope dies with their sibling. It's why many estranged siblings are surprised by the intensity of their own grief, able to acknowledge that their sibling had already been out of their life for a long time, had already been grieved, and yet the finality of estrangement only comes with death.

That same sibling who described herself and her sister as "just different people" went on to recount the experience of losing her as "horrendous. It was the worst thing I have ever experienced. I ended up severely depressed and suicidal. I couldn't breathe or find a reason to go on. I felt her loss in every way. No one understood what it was like. They couldn't understand why I was never 'over it.' I honestly felt that my heart and life had been ripped into shreds." A twin who had lost her brother to suicide explained that "although we were not close, it was shocking, traumatic, and heartbreaking. It changed my life view for a while. The nature of his death (suicide) left me feeling very unsure/insecure about the world around me. The world felt empty and devastating. I felt very angry and I also felt guilty for a long time. I was sad but also frustrated."

Just because you weren't best friends in life does not mean you won't grieve. When it comes to our siblings, that friendship is only one aspect of all that they represent—our childhood, future, genetics, family dynamics, and memories can die along with them. We are left with oh so much more to grieve.

PHYSICAL MANIFESTATIONS OF LOSS

While all our relationships were and are unique, shaped by a nearly infinite combination of factors, the loss of that relationship is a big fucking deal. Regardless of what complexities that relationship held in life, the loss of a sibling is linked to serious physical and mental health outcomes.[8] It is also the least-researched of all forms of familial bereavement. One study on young adult loss compared the loss of a friend to that of a sibling and found that sibling loss is particularly distressing due to the depth of that specific relationship type. Those who lost a sibling expressed higher psychological and physical symptoms than those who lost a friend, including the following:[9]

- Increased likeliness to develop depression and higher levels of depression
- More likely to have complicated grief, with more reported symptoms and severity
- More physical symptoms, with a strong association between level of complicated grief and somatic symptoms (more on that in Chapter 5)
- Significantly lower sense of meaningfulness of the world
- Lower sense of benevolence in the world
- Lower self-worth

I'm going to ask you to go back up and read that list again. Let's just sit on that for a second. Losing a sibling makes you more likely to be depressed and experience complicated grief, have physical symptoms, and significantly less likely to feel a sense of meaningfulness in the world and in ourselves.

You have experienced a significant loss.

It's okay that you are not okay. Your feelings, wherever they fall on the spectrum, are valid. I don't care what anyone else tells you (or doesn't)— your feelings are valid, and your loss is real.

Losing a sibling is, as one brother put it, "profoundly disorienting." We are plunged into a new alternative reality in which family dynamics are shattered, our past and future forever altered beyond recognition, and we are often left to quietly pick up the pieces.

three

The Last Waltz

You can dance, and you can shake. / Things will break, you make mistakes. / You lose your friends, again and again. / 'Cause nothing is ever perfect. / No one's perfect. / Let me say it again, no one's perfect.

—Arcade Fire

I had no idea that April 15, 2009, the day Ben and I took his fiancée's son to see the movie *Monsters vs. Aliens*, would be the last time I'd ever see him. I knew he was getting deployed but didn't know exactly when. This was only supposed to be our last visit before he reported to Fort Dix for training. I was supposed to see him again. This was not supposed to be the end. That summer I was set to travel to Ohio for an internship. I'd pleaded with the director of my graduate program to place me near my family in New York or Connecticut, but those companies were more competitive, and she didn't mince words that my skills were not up to the task. When I found out I'd be in Cleveland I sobbed in the school's hallway surrounded by classmates who knew about my brother's deployment and my desire to be near family. They knew because this was not my first hallway cry.

I'd cried here when I first learned of his deployment and had my first panic attack here when I received a *New York Times* alert about soldiers dead in Afghanistan. I'd been able to call Ben that time. He assured me he'd be okay; he was going to Iraq, which was safer at that time. His advice was to "unsubscribe from *New York Times* alerts, you masochist."

I cried in that hallway when he told me his orders had changed and he'd be going to Afghanistan after all.

There I was, crying in that hallway once again as I suddenly realized I didn't know when I would see my brother again. I didn't know if I'd be able to come home and see him before he deployed. I didn't know if they'd even give him time off before he left. No, I reminded myself, he *will* be coming home. I might not be able to say goodbye before he left, but it wasn't goodbye forever. He promised me it wouldn't be goodbye forever.

Once the worst thing happened, that final visit in April took on a whole new meaning. The visit suddenly had a spotlight on it, my brain screaming, "You must remember every detail of this ordinary day because, as it turns out, that day will matter. A lot." Cool, cool, no pressure. Among those who lost a sibling suddenly, often through violence or fatal accidents, many felt that same spotlight. Combing back through details and grasping for meaning in otherwise ordinary interactions.

One of the strange things about losing Ben suddenly is that people who did have the opportunity to say goodbye, or who treated every visit like it would be their last, would always add some kind of qualifier.

"We saw it coming," said the sister who begged her brother not to leave her alone after his first suicide attempt.

"I *always* gave my brother ten- to twenty-second hugs because I always feared it would be the last," said the sister whose brother had overdosed before.

"He was sick," said the brother who held his dying brother's hand.

"It was an overdose; we always knew it could happen," said the sister left raising her niece.

Watching your sibling suffer is not easier.

Watching them deteriorate, powerless to help, is not easier.

I've heard hundreds of siblings recount their last visit; there is no easier way.

None of this is easy.

MAGICAL FINAL MOMENTS

One thing that struck me throughout my research was the number of siblings who somehow knew to tie up loose ends, even when they didn't see the death coming.

Claudia, whom we met earlier in this chapter, got her first cell phone days before her brother's murder. She called him by mistake while trying to figure out how to use it, and he answered. That was the last time they ever spoke.

Sharae took a picture of her brother alone the last time she saw him. "It was unusual, but somehow I just knew to do it."

In her essay, "David," Elisa Albert writes,

> One night, when you were dying in your hospital bed and I was the only one there with you, I drew the curtains and climbed right into bed beside you. How did I know to do that? I was nineteen years old. I loved you more than I could say. I held you in my arms and rested my head next to yours. You remained unconscious. A machine breathed for you. I held you for a while. I am so, so proud to have done that. To have had that instinct, and to have acted upon it. I don't know how or why, but it made things much easier, later.[1]

Delia Ephron tried to climb into her sister Nora's hospital bed, but there wasn't room with all the tubes she was connected to. "Why don't they have double beds in hospitals?" Delia writes. "If I had a hospital, I'd have double beds in it."[2]

My brother was killed three weeks before his birthday. I'd been assembling a package to mail him, but it was never sent. That package haunted me for years—

What if he died thinking I'd forgotten his birthday?

What if I could have given him one more smile?

What if I could have made him giggle one last time?

My feelings over that unsent package were only the beginning of a postmortem guilt trip unrivaled by even my most guilt-provoking Jewish grandmother. Years after his death I was rereading our emails and stumbled across one I'd sent three days before he died. The last email I ever sent him. He hadn't responded and I forgot I ever sent it.

> Hey Brother!
>
> Sorry I havent been great at writing . . . life got crazy as school picked up and although I think about you 7000 times a day (I've counted), I realize I never tell you that.
>
> In other news, I have 2 DVDs full of movies and the 2nd season of Mad Men to send you. I don't know what else to send because Dad steals all the good package ideas. I'll collect a few things and send it this week. Any requests?
>
> Tufts just passed a rule prohibiting students from performing any sex acts while one's roomate is in the room. Interesting?
>
> How's life there? I can't wait to see you in February!
>
> Love love love love,
>
> A

I have no way of knowing if he even saw it, but a sense of calm washed over me knowing I *did* tell him I loved him that one last time. I told him

I loved him and about the package. I even slipped in a dig at my dad's expense AND a sex joke!

THE DREADED SHOULDS

Guilt from the loss of a sibling is extremely common and uniquely profound due to the nature of sibling relationships.[3] The love/hate, the fighting, the unspoken connections—they all work together to create a Petri dish in which guilt and regret can flourish.

One sibling wrote, "It's the guilt of not being there enough, not doing enough, not loving enough, taking our time for granted; the guilt of knowing she suffered without me; why wasn't it me; the guilt of living my life when she didn't get to live hers."

This is extremely, completely, universally—normal.

Elisabeth Kübler-Ross, a pioneer in the study of death and grief, said, "Guilt is perhaps the most painful companion of death."[4] And isn't it just. As one sibling put it, the loss causes "unique unrest," and what is guilt if not deep, profound, reality-shattering unrest?

I want us to take the time to unpack the most common sources of guilt and remorse that emerged in my research so that you can see the range of experiences and perhaps (if we're lucky) relate to some in a way that will bring you closer to absolution. We will call these . . . drumroll please . . . The Dreaded Shoulds. In talking with other siblings, there was a close connection between the cause of death and/or age at the time of death and The Dreaded Shoulds. In her essay "The Dead-Brother Code Switch," Rachel Sklar perfectly illustrates how the experience of losing a sibling to suicide led to a unique set of Shoulds.

Suicide has an extra dark, heavy layer of awfulness to it, because there's the unavoidable question: Why? Not the unanswerable, inscrutable *why* of "Why me? Why her? Why him? Why us?" that accompanies tragedy that comes without agency. It's the perfectly reasonable question of "But why did he do it?" with a hefty side of "Who missed the signs?" "Who said the wrong thing?" and "Who ought to have known?" It's the unavoidable undercurrent of blame.[5]

Should #1: Should Have Had More Time

The squandered weeks/months/years lost to fights and estrangement. The cruel words said without concern for their impact. The skipped visits. The phone calls, emails, and text messages left unanswered.

All because we assumed we'd have more time. .

When Erika's brother-in-law called, panicked, to say her brother had suffered a heart attack, she could hear the paramedics working on him in the background and all she could think was that they hadn't spoken since they'd had an argument weeks earlier. "Literally my life with my brother flashed through my head. I kid you not. I am not joking. Something in my heart changed. Something in my head sort of broke. All I really remember besides that is I went completely numb."

Others mourned not a specific fight but an ongoing distance. A relationship that was never as close as they'd liked but had the potential to grow if only they had more time.

Not saying "I love you" enough because they took the relationship for granted.

Guilt for what they didn't prioritize when they had the time.

Should #2: Should Have Seen It Coming

We have already established that there is no grass and we are in a mud pit. Within that mud pit, those who did not see the death coming may sift back through every memory looking for moments of foreshadowing. Signs they missed, cries for help that went unanswered, dangers they didn't anticipate.

The surviving sibling who also suffers from depression and believes they should have seen it coming.

The surviving sibling who struggled to connect and carries the guilt that they didn't try harder to understand.

Or me, the sibling convinced her brother would not return from his deployment, torn between the guilt that she somehow *did* see it coming and still couldn't stop it. When I saw it coming, my brother hid the truth. He assured us his unit was the safest one: "We deal with civilians," he'd say. "We're meeting with village leaders, not battling the front lines." While that may have been technically true, it wasn't what it appeared. I know because I spoke to some of his men years later. They knew the dangers.

They saw it coming.

He saw it coming.

He did it anyway.

Should #3: Should Have Done More

When you think you should have seen it coming, it's natural to also think you should have been able to prevent it. In the years after Ben died, my belief that I should have seen it coming led to the guilt that I hadn't done more to stop him. Ben didn't need to go to Afghanistan. He was called up on a stop-loss order to deploy one month *after* his service was up. In his civilian life, he worked for the CDC then FEMA, and he had connections with senators and congressmen—any of these could have been leveraged to clear the order. Would it have been ethical? I honestly couldn't care less.

We tried to convince him not to go. There was no convincing.

"He told me about multiple ways he could have gotten out of it," our brother Sam recounted. "It wasn't about getting out of it. He didn't want to get out of it. He knew what he was doing, and I knew I couldn't convince him."

"Do you feel any guilt," I asked him, "that we didn't try harder to convince him to stay?" Because I sure as shit had been carrying around a mountain of guilt for the past twelve years.

"Guilt?" He sounded almost confused. "No, Annie, no guilt. It seems almost unbelievable that he *wouldn't* have gone. That's just wishful thinking. I know *I* wouldn't have gone, but he was different. We both know the hero's story. When the hero is called to adventure, he must go."

After hanging up the phone my first thought was that I really should have had that conversation with Sam about a decade ago. We had the same conversations with the same person, yet one of us walked away carrying guilt because we didn't do more (even if it was an impossible task) and the other understood, on a deep level, the limitations of their own influence and the power of free will. Maybe that's the manifestation of their love built on admiration.

I thought back on the interviews I'd done with surviving siblings who carried this Dreaded Should, siblings lost to suicide, addiction, and in some cases accidents. Siblings who carried a belief, a conviction even, that we should have been able to predict the future, clear the demons, control fate, save them, save ourselves. Perhaps to clear the guilt we need to come to terms with the powers and limitations of our own influence.

Should #4: Should Have Been Me

Survivor's guilt is a real bitch. Shakespeare doesn't hold a candle to the stories we weave and the alternative scenarios we play out.

In my work, illness was a major trigger of survivor's guilt. For biological siblings, watching their brothers and sisters suffer and succumb to a genetic illness is a unique mind fuck. It is Russian roulette within our genes. It's not just a matter of "it should have been me," but "it just as easily *could* have been me."

Illnesses that aren't genetic elicit a similar guilt. Regardless of the root cause—be it cancer or addiction—you cannot watch this person who is meant to be your longest relationship leave this earth without thinking, "Why them?" and, terrifyingly, "Why not me?"

Why them is a common theme throughout. In the event of a random, sudden, or violent death—such as a homicide or a vehicular accident—the why thems are especially strong. Of all the people in the world, why was mine the one that was taken? But really, it's always someone's person—the guilt is just easier to dismiss when that person isn't ours.

Should #5: Should Be Here

Every new milestone is a shiny new opportunity for guilt. The guilt that you live on and will hit milestones they never did.

For me, the most significant of those milestones have been when I became older than my oldest brother, when I got married, and when I had children. He should have been at my wedding, giving an overly earnest toast as was his way. Instead, my amazing brother Sam had to give a speech on behalf of both of them. Sam, always the comedian, had to fill both roles for his baby sister. He did a phenomenal job—I laughed, I cried, I winced, I cried again—but he shouldn't have needed to do that alone. Ben should have been there.

The Dreaded Shoulds are a natural response to our grief, but ruminating on them can contribute to making us feel "stuck" in our grief. As Claire Bidwell Smith explains in her book *Anxiety: The Missing Stage of Grief*, "Many people try to stop themselves from playing out these alternative scenarios, but really it's just the mind working its way to a level of acceptance."[6] She goes on to stress that releasing the guilt is essential to our own healing and processing, lest it manifest into anger, depression, and anxiety. The only way to do this is by recognizing that these feelings are all rooted in what we think about *ourselves* and the (often unrealistic) expectations and standards we hold ourselves to. Right now, while I'm writing this, I'm listening to the song "Unconditional I (Lookout Kid)" by Arcade Fire. My agent, knowing my obsession with song lyrics, sent it to me a week ago, and I've been listening to it on a loop ever since. Ben would have loved this one. As the words "let me say it again, no one's perfect" repeat in my headphones, I know it's because he wanted to make sure I really heard it.

Here's the thing. That study we talked about in the last chapter—the one that showed high rates of complicated grief in siblings—it also found that conflict within your relationship doesn't change your likelihood of experiencing complicated grief. It's all a mud pit. Let me say it again: no one's perfect.

USING THE SHOULDS

How, then, can we use this guilt—these Shoulds—to get closer to a place of acceptance? And what if this reality is one we have no intention of accepting?

Untangle the Disappointment and Regret.

On the surface, disappointment and regret can feel so very similar, but it is the object of that emotion that truly distinguishes the two. Disappointment is feeling the loss of unmet expectations while acknowledging that the outcome was out of our control. If you expected to spend your entire life with this human, and that time was cut short, you are sure as shit going to feel significantly disappointed. That's okay. Let yourself feel the disappointment without blame. You might also feel disappointment that you never had the sibling relationship you wanted, needed, or deserved. Let yourself mourn the future image painted in your mind and etched into your DNA. Regret is different, though. Regret happens when we *blame ourselves*. Remember those self-beliefs fueling guilt? The very same. Regret isn't necessarily driven by things we did, but often by the things we didn't—those calls we didn't make, visits we never took.

Use It to Do Better.

Both regret and guilt are a function of empathy, and they force us to hold ourselves (and others) to a higher standard in the future. I believe this regret + guilt + empathy connection is the key to getting us closer to a sense of meaning. Feeling guilty that you didn't call enough? Call the amazing people in your life. Regret that you never told them just how much you loved them? Now would be a good time to do that. It's *always* a good time to do that. From time to time, Sam and I will leave each other voicemails or send a quick "I love you!" or "thinking of you!" text message. When I'm really lucky, Sam will leave a voicemail when he's in the car with all four of his kids, in which they'll all be screaming, "I LOVE YOU!"

Forgiving Doesn't Mean Forgetting.

They aren't thinking about those things anymore, so why should you? What a simple concept . . . they aren't thinking about those things anymore. It's time to free yourself from the guilt. Consider this chapter your permission slip; permission to stop carrying that weight, to stop relitigating the past, to focus on the future. This is also your assurance that if you do release that feeling, if you allow yourself to forget your regrets and let go of disappointment, it does not mean you are letting go of your sibling. They do not live on only in your self-loathing, though many would have had you believe that—it's the way siblings are with each other.

Remember the Entirety of Their Lives—Not Only the End.

It's too easy to get fixated on all the things that went wrong, the mistakes and regrets, or to turn the dead into deities. What if instead we remember it all? Not only the good, no reason to create false gods here, but not only the bad either. Breanne lost her brother to suicide when he was only fourteen, an age at which none of us are our best selves, and she explained that she likes to imagine him as an adult, as the person he could have been. Don't immortalize them at their worst, but don't immortalize yourself at your worst either.

four

No New Memories

Always remember there was nothing worth sharing / like the love that let us share our name.

—Avett Brothers

The day my brother died, I was sure there had been a mistake. I maintained, for at least two weeks, that the military had made a grave error. We never got to view the body—how was everyone so sure it was him? Didn't we owe it to him to confirm? It seemed like the least we could do. What if he was still alive out there? Those thoughts weren't rational, I know that now, but I was unable to comprehend a reality in which the Ben I had before October 2, 2009, was the only Ben I'd ever have. There was no future Ben.

It *wasn't* possible. It couldn't be. This was not a world I wanted to exist in. It was the upside down, the twilight zone, the wrong timeline. The new memories I was forming were all amiss.

I remember standing next to Sam as he delivered the eulogy.

I remember his mouth moving, but not the sound that came out.

I remember my eyes scanning the packed sanctuary.

I remember it was a standing-room-only crowd.

I remember Sam made everyone cry—or maybe they were all crying already.

I remember gripping an index card.

I remember taking a calming breath as Sam concluded and handed me the microphone.

I remember asking for memories. More accurately, I remember begging and pleading for them. I asked that people send me memories. I said I'd make them into a book.

Some people did, though not many. I was caught off guard when those emailed memories made things worse. Why did all these strangers know more about my brother than I did? Each note was a reminder of how little I actually knew about his life. I stopped reading them. Project Memory Collection was abandoned.

It was strange how many things *appeared* the same in this new world but were quietly deteriorating under the surface. Our mom, for example, had long been collecting sea glass on her morning walks along the shoreline. Over the years she has amassed a large collection of beautiful translucent vessels that overflow with smooth, colorful glass treasures. After Ben died, without telling anyone, she labeled which vessels were found when he was alive. That way, she later told me, she'd always know which were found in that part of her life—some found by his very hands. A physical representation of the memories that stopped on October 2, 2009. She has added more overflowing sea glass vessels to her collection in the decade-plus since Ben's death, but the one she was filling at the time of his death remains only half full. Stunted. When, years after Ben's death, my toddler tried to put a new piece of sea glass in that half-filled vessel, I dove to stop him with the same urgency I would if he'd been reaching for a lit flame. The two collections were never to be combined.

You might have moments like this too. Books, movies, songs, even entire rooms that are off-limits in your grief. That's okay. You've experienced a significant loss, and you can't just muscle your way through it.

In his book *The Art of Making Memories*, Meik Wiking describes memories as the "glue that allows us to understand and experience being the same person over time."[1] Except, how can I be the same person over time if I spent twenty-five years as a younger sister with two older brothers—and I was now expected to live the remainder of my life without one of them? There was a crack in the glue. Instead of having one big collection of sea glass, I'd have two smaller ones—one found in a world that no longer exists.

Wiking goes on to explain that memories are our "superpower which allows us to travel in time and sets us free from the limitations of the present moment."[2] When I read that I thought of the sea glass and questioned its logic for the first time. Ben wasn't there on the beach when my mom filled up a vessel of sea glass in 2010, but he *was* present. My mom was likely thinking of him as she combed the beach, his name has been invoked around it, and the pieces bear a striking resemblance to those he'd found a year earlier. Why can't they mix? What if memories, like the trajectory of our lives, aren't linear? What if memories are our key to time travel?

MEMORIES AND IMAGINATION

Memories are built from past experiences—lessons learned, experiences lived—but have you ever felt like you held a memory of the future? Those visions of what is still to come; the daydreams that feel like foregone conclusions. How many times have you second-guessed yourself, unsure of whether a conversation happened out loud or if you'd just thought about it, confusing memory from fantasy? In this way, memory and imagination are very similar neurological processes both housed in the hippocampus. Past research has shown, for example, that people with amnesia who struggle to access their memory also struggle to imagine the future. Those visions of our future are based on the foundation of memory that taught us how similar events tend to unfold, overlaid with the new and novel fantasy of the future. For many of us every life stage, milestone, and event we've experienced in our lives has been with this other person. They are at the foundation of both our memory and our imagination.

I knew (assumed?) I would reach the age of thirty-three, but I never imagined that turning thirty-three would make me older than my oldest brother. That would have been impossible based on the memories that all future birthday visions were built upon. And so, the year I became older than my oldest brother I tried to skip my birthday completely. Was that a healthy, mature response? I honestly don't care. It was what I needed to reconcile my memory from my reality. I removed my birthdate from Facebook in hopes of people forgetting. It felt overly dramatic, but I just did not want to be celebrating. While the intensity of grief may decrease over time, reaching milestones your sibling never hit remains traumatic throughout adulthood. The more I talked with other grieving siblings, the more I realized that this kind of reaction wasn't dramatic or unusual at all, that I wasn't alone.

Elizabeth lost her older brother twenty-six years ago, and yet she can still remember those firsts as if they just happened. "My brother and I had the same birthday month. He turned a year older first, and ten days later was my birthday," she explained. "Six months after his death when that month came around, I had a panic attack and thought, 'Since he won't be turning a year older, then neither could I.' It was so strong it felt like my blood was running cold in me. I was sitting at Chuck E. Cheese and my kids were playing and lots of families were around when this hit. It scared me."

Each year, as we move through milestones—many of which our siblings will never experience—our lives veer slightly off the course we'd always imagined; the new memories feel warped and misaligned with our vision for them. I never even considered the fact that my brother might not be at my wedding. That he might never meet my children or have his own. And yet, every year I step deeper and deeper into the future he never had, collecting memories we should have shared.

SIBLINGS' SHARED MEMORY

I often wondered, in those early days, if the remainder of my life would include an obvious void. I knew I would *feel* the absence of his presence, but would other people be able to see it? Would future photos have a blank space where Ben should be? Would my memories contain that same hole? I couldn't imagine how that would work—the logistics of it. Would my memories shrink to fit a family of four, rather than its previous five? Rob recounted how, after his sister died by suicide, "I couldn't compartmentalize her as only existing in one phase of my life." That was when I realized my conviction that Ben wasn't dead those first few weeks was because my brain could not compartmentalize and comprehend the fact that he would only (physically) exist in one phase of my life. Siblings I surveyed articulated this phenomenon so succinctly in their responses:

"It's a never-ending, consistent void that permeates your existence."

"The silence is gut-wrenching."

"I am indescribably lonely."

No matter what the relationship—wonderful, very close, fraught, even estranged—siblings are often the only other people on earth who know our childhoods almost as well as we do. When you have a sibling, there's always a backup memory; someone you can consult when your memory gets cloudy, someone to fill those gaps and be the glue. This was a consistent sentiment regardless of how close that relationship was. You might not have wanted them there, but in childhood you were forced together regardless. Remember, in childhood siblings spend more time alone together than with their parents; that's a lot of shared memory.

Ben's memory could be used to sharpen my fuzziest recollections and fill in those early years before my memory formed. He surely remembered more of my early life than I did. Was that gone too? One surveyed sibling wrote, "Losing a sibling is like losing part of your childhood, and all the memories you had growing up with that person that no one else knows about seem lost and gone forever." Another wrote, "It feels like my childhood memories are gone. I have no one to confirm them with, to reminisce with."

I am extremely fortunate that Ben did leave me many of those memories, captured in diaries left behind on a shelf in our parents' home. Diaries I didn't open for nearly a decade, filled with detailed accounts of our family dynamics, speculation on the future of his younger siblings, and even one entry from the day I was born. Did they answer every question I had? No, of course not. Were they full of insightful Indigo Girls lyrics? Yes, of course they were. They've become my most prized possession, and I feel eternally lucky that he kept them so diligently. One thing I've learned from the existence of those diaries is to just write it down. Ironic, perhaps, that Ben's persistent advice for me whenever I'd call him with a problem or complaint was to "write it down," and I resisted with all my might. I did not want to write it down; I wanted him to tell me our parents were too strict, I was always right, and that I would one day become a powerful queen who could imprison her middle school bullies with a flick of her wrist. *Was that really so much to ask, Ben?!* But I digress . . .

MEMORY CONFORMITY

Depending on someone else's memory to confirm our own can be comforting—or at the very least, supporting—but it is one of the reasons why people so often misremember firsthand experiences and have clear memories of moments we've only heard about in stories. Like the story of Ben daring Sam to punch his stomach after a large meal and the projectile vomit that sprang forth when the little brother eagerly took the bait. I'm not sure I'd even been born yet, but I have heard that story enough times to have created a full visual episodic memory of it. My memory conformed to the stories I'd heard.

Memory conformity is when another person's memory informs your own. It's how we "remember" things that never happened to us; it's why I can still imagine myself standing next to Sam as he landed that fateful blow on Ben's bloated gut. It's yet another way in which our memory and our imagination are intrinsically linked.

A 2009 study conducted by Elin Skagerberg and Daniel Wright sought to explore the concept of memory conformity by studying sibling pairs. The idea was that since humans validate their memories via comparison to others, who better to compare yourself to than your longest relationship? Researchers hypothesized that older siblings would hold more power in the relationship and younger siblings would disproportionately conform to their older siblings' memory. I would have held the same hypothesis myself. It felt much more likely that I would conform to my brothers' memories and not the other way around.

As a researcher, my favorite studies are those that disprove a seemingly logical hypothesis, and this one did not disappoint.

The study found that, yes, older siblings did tend to hold more power and make the majority of decisions, but younger siblings did *not* disproportionately conform to the memories of the older. It was much more poetic than that. Memory conformity depends not on power but on the strength of the social bond. It was the *balance* of power. The stronger the bond between the siblings, the more they conformed their memory to each other's, and trust was the key to memory accuracy; the more they trusted their siblings, the more accurate respondents' own memories were.[3]

These shared memories aren't dictated by birth order; they're cultivated through strong connections and mutual trust.

MEMORY SPECTRUM

Memories can be terrifying, illusive, precious, and chaotic; so why can't we let them remain preserved in the past? Why is it important that we excavate our past?

Put simply—the view we hold of our own past matters. It's why nostalgia sells and *Gilmore Girls* got a reboot. Studies have shown that holding a positive view of the past makes people happier in the future. Therein lies a key to our future survival in this new world. According to Wiking, "Long term happiness can depend on the ability to form a positive narrative of the past."[4] That positive nostalgia boosts our self-esteem and heightens our feelings of *being* loved—it is a form of self-protection.

However, nostalgia is not inherently a productive or healthy emotion; it was initially regarded as a disease with symptoms that included "loss of appetite, fainting, heightened suicide risk, and hallucinations of the people and places you miss."[5] In order to feel nostalgia, we place ourselves at the center of our narrative memory in a way that might not be reflective of reality.

In that way, nostalgia can be both beneficial and detrimental to our psyche, depending on how we reconstruct the past. It is important that we not shy away from these memories—the good, the bad, and the mysterious—as they're essential records of our own identities. Making sense of them is fundamental to our future, but we must do so with care and integrity.

Once someone is gone, the realization that there will be no new memories puts even more pressure on those we *do* have. Remember in the '90s when everyone was collecting Beanie Babies, and then one day they became rare and valuable and suddenly Patti the Platypus was valued at $20,000? Our memories are those rare Beanie Babies—once so common-place they were included with your Happy Meal, now rare and valuable enough to end friendships and marriages. We put them in glass cases, no longer willing to let our children play with them or our friends borrow them because they mean too much—they're worth too much. But we must use those memories, for, as emotions expert George A. Bonanno says in *The Other Side of Sadness*, "the accuracy of our memories does not determine how we grieve; that is determined by what we do without memories, how we experience them, and what we take from them during bereavement."[6]

Our memories are inextricably linked to the relationship we have with the people in those memories, as the quality of the relationship often dictates that of the memory. Those relationship factors we discussed in Chapter 2? They come back to haunt us in our memories. Good, bad, invisible, or ugly—let's explore them all.

THE GOOD

Kim was the one to plan her brother's funeral, and when I asked about the weight of that responsibility, she immediately jumped to point out her other siblings' involvement and that, unbelievably, it wasn't all bad. The night before the funeral, she described, "We [siblings] stayed up creating the slideshow and, like, laughed and had a good time. It . . . " She paused. "It wasn't all just the drudgery of it. And it felt better to do something and be productive." That simple act of allowing themselves to find joy in memory while assembling the slideshow is much more difficult than it may seem on paper, as it requires us to hold both pain and joy at the same time. These emotional contradictions reside at the core of what it means to be human; but that doesn't make it easy.

Then there are the positive memories that carry guilt or pain along with them. The guilt that you shouldn't feel levity or joy. The limiting belief that you do not deserve to be happy. The (false) belief that being happy means you're okay with what happened. Others carry with them the painful reminder that those moments will live in the past forever, with no possibility for similar memories to be created in the future. "Remember that time we went to dinner" can quickly turn to "we'll never eat a meal together again," and then, within our minds and hearts, all hell breaks loose.

When I spoke with Cara, she shared that she often tries to forget the painful memories surrounding her brother and the lost potential in their relationship because remembering triggers guilt. I noticed that every memory she recounted revolved around her brother's death. Couched in about a thousand disclaimers about not being a therapist myself, I pointed out what I'd observed and asked, "What if you focused more on his life? And on that relationship? Does that feel like something that you would *want* to do?"

I could see the emotions run across her face, a moment of defensiveness turned quickly to thoughtfulness, then relief, and then . . . a smile. "I had never thought about it that way?" she responded as if it were a question. "You're right, I do default to that super traumatic day and how awful that was. I've never thought about really focusing on his life and celebrating that instead of just . . . " she paused, collecting herself, "it always seems so heavy and dark that I just don't want to think about it. But that makes so much sense—why would I focus on that? Why not focus on the happier side? Or at least try to remember some of those happier memories?"

There's a unique kind of desperation that arises when positive memories seem completely inaccessible. Bonanno explains that

> The bereaved people who are able to deal with a loved one's death, and who are able to accept the finality of the loss, are also able to find comfort in memories of that person. . . . In contrast, other bereaved people, those who are more debilitated by loss, find it harder to hold onto positive memories, as if they can no longer find the person they lost, as if the memories are hidden from them. The pain of grief, it seems, can block all memories of the good.[7]

Take a moment to reread that. When we cannot access those memories, we can no longer find our person. You know the memories are there, but you're unable to conjure them on command. It's like when someone asks your favorite song and you immediately forget every piece of music you've ever heard and cannot think of a single song title. Those moments, when our minds go blank, can be terrifying.

What if I've forgotten forever?

Those memories are all I have.

Excavating those positive memories is worth it, I promise. Remembering and feeling joy doesn't mean you don't still grieve; it simply means you're learning to hold joy and pain at the same time. To those bereaved people who are able to deal with the death, Bonanno explains,

> They know their loved one is gone, but when they think and talk about the deceased, they find that they haven't lost everything. The *relationship* isn't completely gone. They can still call to mind and find joy in the positive shared experiences. It is as if some part of their relationship is still alive.[8]

I suppose that's because it is . . . Memory is alive, and it allows us to hop in that time machine and keep our loved ones alive too.

Meik Wiking's Happiness Research Institute conducted a 2018 study across seventy-five countries in which they asked respondents to describe a happy memory and rate their own happiness. They found a correlation between the number of words used to describe the happy memory and the current happiness level of the memory holder.[9] The more we dive into our positive memories, the happier we feel in that moment. The more we embrace those happy memories, the more *alive* our relationship remains.

Writing this chapter has been extremely emotionally challenging for me because I find myself slipping back into the void over and over again just as I attempt to climb out of it. Turns out, writing about the lack of new memories doesn't help—not in the way remembering positive memories does. And so, I've been trying something new: Each time I find myself slipping (or crying in the bathroom of Madison Coffee House like I am now), I lean into the memories. I close my eyes and try to remember the sound of his high-pitched giggle, look at photos of us smiling together, or listen to one of his favorite songs. I try to use the positive memories to remind myself that our relationship is alive, that a piece of him remains. And it works . . . at least for now.

Promise me you will at least try to feel the happy, dear reader. If you're one of the lucky ones, fortunate enough to have positive memories of your sibling (which is not a given, by any means), then it is your duty, under Sibling Code 156.10.143, to celebrate it *in full*. Not only will it help you keep your sibling's memory alive, but it will bring you joy.

THE BAD

Our society often dismisses the experience of mourners who are grieving imperfect people and imperfect relationships. A fraught or distant relationship in life can result in an even more diminished response to grief, full of unhelpful comments like "I didn't think you two were close" or "this must be a relief." And yes, as we know, sometimes it *is* a relief, but no one else is allowed to tell you that. That's for you, and you alone, to decide.

For some siblings, there aren't many or any good memories. We need to acknowledge and make space for that.

THE INVISIBLE

In analyzing responses to my own sibling loss study, I'm ashamed to admit that I was surprised by the number of responses from people who lost siblings they'd never met or had no memory of. Brothers and sisters lost at birth, in infancy, or born and gone before the surviving sibling was even born. Curious to understand more, I explored the work of Diane Kempson and Vicki Murdock at the University of Wyoming, who studied the impact of "siblings never known" on surviving adult siblings. Too young to fully process the loss, these siblings were not involved in the grieving process, resulting in "unresolved or lifelong grief." While they didn't hold their own first-person memories, these surviving siblings showed a tremendous amount of care and value in keeping their sibling's memory alive. Of the fifteen siblings involved in the study, twelve of them were the "primary memory keeper" within their families for the deceased sibling. In the words of one forty-six-year-old respondent, "I'm probably the one that's the least willing to let her be forgotten." Many report having a continued relationship with their siblings: speaking to them, imagining what they'd be like, and feeling a sense of yearning for the lost relationship. Those are memories too, in their own way, and those memories matter.[10]

You don't need to remember your sibling to understand their impact. The death of a child inevitably alters the family structure and dynamic—and in this case it is perhaps the single most influential contributor to the familial dynamic in which surviving siblings are raised.

DELAYED MEMORIES

"Suddenly at the very moment when, so far, I mourned H least, I remembered her best. Indeed it was something almost better than memory; an instantaneous, unanswerable impression. To say it was like a meeting would be going too far. Yet there was that in it which tempts one to use those words. It was as if the lifting of the sorrow removed a barrier . . . and the remarkable thing is that since I stopped bothering about it, she seems to meet me everywhere."

—C. S. Lewis, *A Grief Observed*

There's a unique kind of shock when a new memory surfaces years later. Sometimes it's a good revelation—other times . . . not so much. Kyle was surprised by the "spark of memory" that would overcome him in an instant and make him cry. That's the thing about memories, they tend to just pop up. A smell will trigger a memory you haven't thought of in years; a revelation will poke its head out like whack-a-mole when you least expect it. With time, many memories may become hazy and lose their details, but as a result, those that do emerge may feel stronger than ever. Some carry more joy—others more pain. I wish I could summon them on command, but so far I struggle to control the timing of their appearance.

Common Scenario One:
Me: Hey, brain, I haven't had a new memory of Ben in a while and I miss him, can you send me one? Maybe I can dream of him tonight?
Brain: One work-related anxiety dream, coming right up!

Common Scenario Two:
Me: Hey, brain, I'm at a really important work event and don't want to end up crying in the bathroom while my coworkers pretend not to notice. Can you please keep it together?
Brain: OMG do you remember that time your brother died?

And away we go.
Delayed memories might not be the most convenient, but sometimes they're the thing we need, or at least they're the thing we get; so it's best to brace yourself and be open to them. It might be the most real feeling of memory we get.

MEMORY COLLECTIVE

Our siblings' friends hold a piece of them that we may have never known. I was ten when Ben graduated high school. I'm not the one who holds his teenage memories. Sure, I'd heard anecdotes and high-lights over the years, but I can't say I truly *knew* teenage Ben. Most of those memories live in the minds of his best friends. I yearned for those stories—to know who he was throughout his life and fill my world with new stories of him. Perhaps asking for memories at the funeral was simply too early for me. Some part of me knew I'd need those memories one day, but I hadn't been ready yet. Now I knew all I wanted was to talk to his friends—the four boys whose voices I'd hear spilling out of Ben's room, who were kind to me and filled our home with teenage giggles. Unfortunately, they wouldn't want to hear from me, I was convinced. I am the annoying baby sister; I am the living reminder that their fifth is dead.

The more time passed, the more comfortable I became with the idea of mining their memories. That's why, in the months leading up to the ten-year anniversary of Ben's death, I emailed them and asked if they'd share their memories. Not only did they say yes, but I learned that they'd been yearning for that same connection and were afraid that reaching out would be triggering. One by one, I interviewed them, recorder in hand, and collected their memories. I was the memory keeper, and they were relieved to no longer be the sole owners and protectors of this piece of Ben. They had been simultaneously afraid of forgetting and not wanting to burden the family with their memories.

It wasn't until two years after those interviews—two years in which we all kept in touch, visited each other, and shared our memories—that I spoke to Claire Bidwell Smith. You know what her advice was? To go back and research your story. Talk to other people and be sure your narrative is correct because it is easy (and human) to misremember. Good memories or bad, creating that narrative of ourselves is an essential step to understanding our own identity. By that time, I had no doubt that reconnecting with Ben's Boys™ was the right thing to do, that it had helped heal a crack within me and brought a piece of Ben back to life, but it was that conversation that allowed me to understand exactly *why*. The narrative that I'd created, with their help, had allowed me to both understand my own identity and fuel my time machine.

five

The Uniqueness of Grief

Give me hope / that emptiness brings fullness / and loss of love brings wholeness to us all.

—Indigo Girls

Every culture approaches grief and mourning differently; broadly construed, there's been a shift in the West. In many ways we've become desensitized—or assumed to be—with death all around us, whether it's the 2010 earthquake in Haiti that caused 160,000 deaths or the 48,117 people killed by guns in the US in 2022 alone. It becomes incomprehensible. And it seems we now live in a world where the bereaved are expected to return to normal, and grieving any longer than your employer's "generous" five-day bereavement leave equates to failure and weakness. This faulty belief has left many unmoored when faced with the wound of grief that may scab over but will never fully heal.

Victorians made sure everyone around you knew you were grieving with a prescribed wardrobe and strict rules for engaging in society. Do I want to return to a period in which culture dictated exactly what I wore and for how long? No, of course not. But what I deeply appreciate, and respect, is the clear understanding that grief takes time. That it is something you live with; that life doesn't just return to normal after the funeral; that sometimes you cannot verbally express your emotions but you can wear them; that grief is something to be acknowledged and incorporated into everyday life.

Only in recent history has Western society begun to acknowledge grief's lifelong hold on us. Not the Victorian *practice* of mourning (we're not dictating fashion here), but the understanding that grief is forever. As Sarah said of her sister's death, "It's for life. I will grieve her for the rest of my life until I see her again."

I often return to the idea of Victorian mourning jewelry. These beautiful heirloom pieces made of dark stones, cameos, or lockets, inlaid with hair from the deceased. At first I thought it was a dark and disturbing tradition. Why do I want a dead person's hair on my finger or around my neck? But the more comfortable I become with my own grief, the more I fall in love with the tradition. It's a visible sign of our loss, one that deserves to be seen. It's a talisman.

We've gone from wearing black for years adorned with locks of our loved one's hair inlaid in heirloom jewelry to packing away their belongings and returning to work the day after their funeral and just . . . moving on. But HOW? How the hell do we move on? That's what I could not wrap my head around early in my grief. How and why; because even if I could figure out how to live without Ben, I didn't want to.

It's undeniable that damage has been done to all of us by the notion that grief can be healed and fixed. It cannot. So instead of trying, and failing, to make it go away, let's learn how to live with it, among it, beside it.

No, mourning is not a recipe to follow. It is a complete rewrite of the recipe for our lives. But it's *your* recipe and you own it—its ingredients, steps, all of it. It's time to get really specific about our grief and what does (and does not) help us work through our own individual experiences, and how to build an effective vocabulary to express those needs.

How will we do this?

I'm so glad you asked. All of the activities in Part II work together to create a comprehensive Mourner's User Manual.

But, Annie, I don't read user manuals.

Correct, no one does. But if you choose to write this one, and even if you never read it again, that will be enough.

WRITING YOUR MANUAL

There would have been no way to write your MUM before your loss. Even if you saw it coming, if you'd been preparing yourself for weeks, months, years, there is no way to anticipate what you will feel once your sibling is gone. In that way, grief is similar to becoming a parent or falling in love; there is no way to anticipate the depth of emotion, or your physical and emotional reaction to it, until it happens to you. No amount of reading, preparing, anticipating, or hearing the experiences of others can fully prepare you for deep grief. This is partly because each loss is unique, and thus each evokes emotions we've never experienced, and partly because we each grieve a little differently. This is beautiful, in a way—a very distant, beautiful-in-theory way. In practice it makes everything that much more complicated. If we all grieved the same, it would be a lot easier to help and understand one another. It would be easier to understand ourselves.

I find comfort in the act of sitting by my brother's grave. I don't think he's actually there, and I don't need to be at the grave to feel his presence, but sometimes I need to just throw myself 1,000 percent into the Dead Brother Experience (DBE™) so that I can move through it.

My brother Sam doesn't need to visit the cemetery to process his grief. When I asked him about it in those first painful years after Ben's death, he explained simply, "I don't think he's there; I don't think visiting the cemetery is visiting Ben. It's just not helpful for me."

It's just not helpful for me.

In my research, it became evident early on that each sibling I spoke to had at least one thing—reaction, struggle, tradition—that they thought was "abnormal" or "wrong." Not a single one of those confessions was one I hadn't heard of in previous interviews, read about in the grief literature, or experienced myself.

Sharae warned me at the beginning of our interview that she probably wouldn't cry. What struck me was that she felt the need to give a disclaimer. On the one hand, great that she knows herself and is okay with how she grieves—but how many times was her grief misunderstood before she started explaining herself to others? "I don't do a lot of crying," she went on, "but that doesn't mean I'm not sad."

So why the shame? Why the self-doubt? I believe it's because we don't actually make space for unique grief. Each person and relationship is unique, so why would our grief not follow suit?

The beautiful-in-theoryness of unique grief can leave us unable to relate to other mourners. The (false) narrative that there is a right way to mourn would also then dictate that there is a wrong way. But that's the thing—there is no wrong way! Acknowledging the uniqueness of grief and learning what does—and does not—work for you is essential to owning the loss as your own. As one sibling put it, "I wish people knew that my experience was unique and needed to be allowed to exist and breathe without having to look like anyone else's grief. I felt that my pain was hugely ignored and overlooked as the sibling."

FORMS OF GRIEF

Grief is a broad term, like "cancer" or "cheese." It defines the general vicinity of your emotions, but it isn't nearly specific enough to truly understand it. Because grief, like love, is felt and expressed differently for every individual. Did you know there are over fifteen commonly understood forms of grief? And did you know they're not mutually exclusive? So many opportunities for nuanced grief! I'll take one order of complicated grief with a side of disenfranchised grief and anticipatory grief sprinkled on top, please!

Here's a quick overview of some common forms[1] of grief:[2]

- **Normal or Resilient Grief** (I'm not okay, but I will be.)

  This is an extremely misleading term in that all forms of grief are "normal" grief, but in this case "normal grief" refers to the process in which the bereaved can address and process the loss in a way that allows them to grow through it toward a place of acceptance. There is still anger, despair, shock, crying, etc., but there is also progress.
- **Anticipatory Grief** (Death is imminent.)

  This is a grief and mourning that begins before the death has taken place, but its inevitability is known. This is most common if the deceased was ill or struggled with addiction and/or mental health issues. It's also the grief you feel in anticipation of milestones or events related to the deceased.
- **Complicated Grief a.k.a. Prolonged Grief Disorder** (A fixation on grief.)

  Complicated grief is a form of prolonged and intensified grief that often includes difficulty accepting the loss, preoccupation with the circumstances surrounding it, and a painful combination of bitterness, anger, yearning, and intense longing.[3]
- **Chronic Grief** (Grief that doesn't get any easier.)

  An experience of grief in which the intensity of your grief in the immediate aftermath of loss does not subside over time, and instead intensifies.
- **Delayed Grief** (Grief? What grief?)

  This is grief's snooze button, kicking the can down the ol' grief road for years. Delayed grief is grief experienced years after the loss, as it was not processed as it should have been initially.

- **Distorted Grief** (In which the grief takes on a physical form.)

  In distorted grief, the bereaved experiences an extreme reaction to the loss and it changes their overall behavior; namely, you see increased self-destructive behavior.
- **Cumulative Grief** (When bad things come in multiples.)

  Cumulative grief is when the hits just keep coming, and you experience a second loss while still deeply grieving the first.
- **Exaggerated Grief** (Grief on steroids.)

  Exaggerated grief manifests in excessive or disruptive behavior, substance abuse, abnormal fears, and nightmares. It is more exaggerated than distorted grief and can lead to thoughts of suicide or self-harm and, in some cases, the emergence of a psychiatric disorder.
- **Secondary Loss** (The domino effect.)

  All of the subsequent losses that you experience as a result of the central loss: your children losing the opportunity for a relationship with their aunt or uncle, the loss of your nuclear family as you knew it. Each of these secondary losses becomes a new loss of its own. *(More on this in Chapter 10.)*
- **Masked Grief** (Grief that doesn't look like grief.)

  Grief that is hidden so well, and so deeply, that even the bereaved doesn't believe they are grieving. This can manifest in physical ailments and issues, most of which seem completely unrelated to the loss but are actually caused by the emotional suppression.
- **Disenfranchised Grief** (Grief that isn't recognized.)

  The grief that isn't validated or given the space to be expressed. This is most often because your community, culture, or society doesn't recognize your loss or the weight of it. This could be because of your relationship with the deceased or their cause of death.
- **Traumatic Grief** (The grief + PTSD cocktail.)

  This type of grief is most common among those who experienced a sudden, violent, or unexpected loss, those who experienced trauma in childhood, and those whose siblings suffered physically.

- **Collective Grief** (The grief that binds us together.)

  It is New York City coming together after 9/11 and New Orleans after Hurricane Katrina. Collective grief is experienced by an entire community.

- **Inhibited Grief** (The "I'm fine" grief.)

  Those experiencing inhibited grief give no outward indication of their grief; instead, they hold it in and restrain it. This inability to move through grief can lead to physical reactions.

- **Abbreviated Grief** (Short grief.)

  Abbreviated grief is just that—it doesn't last as long as it might otherwise, and the bereaved is able to move forward shortly after the loss. This could be due to a weak emotional attachment or extended illness of the deceased.

- **Absent Grief** (Grief? You in there?)

  Absent grief is . . . gone. There are no physical signs of grief beyond the initial shock and disbelief.

While we all might identify with one or more of these forms of grief, I want us to focus on those that are most pervasive among bereaved siblings. Unfortunately, many of those are also the least acknowledged and understood, so it's even more essential that we discuss them.

NORMAL OR RESILIENT GRIEF

No form of grief is "easy," and each loss is experienced uniquely, which can make "normal grief" seem like an oversimplification of a tremendously complex emotion. I struggled to wrap my head around the concept, as well, because how can losing a sibling be normal? In recent years, some experts have begun to refer to this as "resilient grief," which, I'll admit, seems a bit more accurate. Normal grief isn't easy, it's not simple, and it's not cookie-cutter—but it is resilient. Those who experience it are able to grieve, process, and grow over time without getting stuck in the muck. I think of resilient grief as a grief with forward momentum—the bereaved makes progress in their processing of the loss, and they are able to find meaning and purpose in their own lives moving forward. In many ways, this form of grief lives in the absence of all others. It's a grief experienced *without* stagnation, PTSD, inhibition, or the many other characteristics that define the other grief types on our list.

When I spoke to siblings who exhibited resilient grief, I couldn't help but feel a sense of awe. How did they know it would be okay? How were they able to get to this place of peace so much earlier than I could? How did they have this . . . this confidence in the universe? Rob was one of the first siblings I spoke to who embodied this resilience, and I kept trying to understand how he did it. There was no question that he loved his sister deeply and unconditionally, and it was obvious that her death had torn his world apart, and yet he was able to remain positive. "When it happened, the only way forward for me was to find some of the positives," he explained. "I needed to hold on to them and grow them. Because there are positives that you can hold on to, and I'd rather spend my time focused on the very, very limited positives than the plentiful negatives. It was very clear to me at an early stage in my grief that there were two paths to go down. And I felt comfortable embracing the positive path."

If your brain works like Rob's, and you saw those paths and chose the positive one—I commend you. For whatever reason, my brain only saw one option, and I wish that hadn't been the case. Following that positive path doesn't mean you're okay with the loss or that you wouldn't change it if you could; to be resilient in your grief means that you're able to accept the reality you're facing, and adapt to it.

COMPLICATED GRIEF A.K.A. PROLONGED GRIEF DISORDER

If you've never heard of complicated grief, you're not alone.

Complicated grief can be characterized as prolonged and intensified grief that often includes difficulty accepting the loss, preoccupation with the circumstances surrounding it, and a painful combination of bitterness, anger, yearning, and longing.[4] Some studies have also found that complicated grief leads to increased rates of estrangement, intrusive thoughts, and psychological distress at symbolic events.

For me, it was the intrusive thoughts. My conviction that I would lose my son because my mother had lost her firstborn. Never mind that my son was two and, as my therapist pointed out at the time, not in an active war zone like my brother was. But logic couldn't penetrate the depth of my conviction. It wasn't only that I feared it, it was that I was convinced of its inevitability.

In Dorothy P. Holinger's *The Anatomy of Grief*, she provides perhaps the best and most succinct summary: "Complicated grief is relentless."[5] Complicated grief intrudes and works its way into every thought, every moment, every cell. That preoccupation and relentless yearning does not diminish over time; its intensity can last for years.

Years out from their sibling's death, some siblings I spoke with were beginning to see the real-life impact of their complicated grief transpire and only then realized anything was amiss. Parents who had worked through their grief in a way that seemed impossible were now able to talk about their lost child with joy and peace, whereas siblings couldn't even say their names without crying.

While anyone can experience complicated grief following a loss, there are some factors that seem to make it more likely. These include the closeness or depth of relationship to the person who died, lack of support, stress, and a predisposition to depression and anxiety. In Chapter 2, we touched on a study that explored complicated grief in young adults grieving a sibling compared to those grieving a friend. That study found that a whopping 57 percent of bereaved young adult siblings expressed symptoms of complicated grief, versus 15 percent of those grieving a friend.[6] It is estimated that 7–10 percent of bereaved in the US experience complicated grief, so that 57 percent is a big deal.

When I first read that study, I was in my late thirties, and I started reading it with the mind of a researcher—digging for all the information that could be relevant and helpful in the writing of this book. But as I read, all I could think about was twenty-five-year-old Annie, that young adult on the precipice of life who watched that life crumble around her like a scene in a horror movie. I feel so deeply for that Annie; she didn't even have a chance. That Annie, like many young adults, was setting up her life. Imagine carefully setting up bowling pins in formation: job, apartment, friends, dating, graduate school, all balanced precariously but balanced nonetheless. Then a bowling ball smashes into them, shattering the formation and sending pins flying in the air. But some pins are broken, they can't be set up again, and you don't have enough experience (in bowling or in life) to repair and reset the pins.

Complicated grief is real, and it has the very real ability to impact every aspect of our existence, making it difficult to participate in everyday life and leading to increased isolation of the bereaved. Because of the intensity and relentless persistence of complicated grief, along with the intense impact it can have on all aspects of our lives (on top of the impact of the loss itself), professional treatment is strongly advised. And while we will continue to discuss and unpack complicated grief throughout this book, that does not constitute professional treatment, as I am not a therapist and this is not a customized treatment. I know that finding a therapist can be a daunting task, but it doesn't have to be. Start by visiting PsychologyToday.com, and on the top of the page you'll see "find a therapist"—enter your zip code and just read through the bios you find. Look for someone who specializes in grief. If that feels like too much, consider enlisting a good friend to do the initial search for you and generate a few suggestions. Give that same friend some availabilities and let them schedule for you. Your friends *want* to help. This is a moment when you can let them.

DISENFRANCHISED GRIEF

Disenfranchised losses are those that are trivialized by society and those around us. Multiple studies have shown higher-than-average rates of disenfranchised grief among surviving siblings, and as a result, siblings didn't get the support, validation, and help they needed. Disenfranchised grief isn't harmless and the mourner experiencing it isn't being selfish or needy. The lack of social and emotional support that results from disenfranchised grief has real-world implications for the bereaved, including increased rates of avoidant coping and complicated grief.[7]

The thing I find most infuriating about disenfranchised grief is that it can feel like the world is telling you there is only a finite amount of grief to go around. That you grieving less somehow allows others to grieve more. It does not. Grief is not a finite resource to be rationed. Just as finishing your own meal will not magically feed starving children in other countries, allowing siblings to grieve does not diminish the loss of any other. As one sibling reflected, "Diminishing one's pain and grief for another's is cruel."

Remember Kenny? He's the one who spoke to his brother every morning on their way to work as they flipped each other off on the freeway. The first time anyone checked up on him—only him—was more than six months after his brother's death. Until then, he hadn't realized that no one had reached out and asked how he was doing; once one person did, it put the previous six months into stark relief. "It took him calling me before I realized no one's called to just check up on me." Kenny admitted that he doesn't think he'd have known to reach out to a friend if the roles had been reversed; and so there was no anger, no resentment, no placing of blame. But there was sadness in the isolation and in the reminder that the person who checked in on him every morning on his way to work was gone.

Another sibling had a similar experience except the call was from her father, who reached out six months after their loss with a revelation: "I just realized you lost someone also," he said. "How are you?"

For those who did not have a positive or public relationship with their siblings in life, disenfranchised grief can be even more pronounced. Those grieving siblings told me they felt like they weren't supposed to grieve as much as they were; but you don't need to be close to feel the pain. Your life and family are still forever altered. The person who shared your most formative years is still gone. Your future is still forever altered.

I invite you to take a second now and close your eyes. Wait, no—read this next part and *then* close your eyes. This will be easier in the audiobook. Let's try again. Think about all the times you have felt like your grief was disenfranchised. The times someone asked about your family but never asked about you. The times your loss was shrugged off due to your sibling's cause of death (more on this in Chapter 7) or your outward relationship with them. Okay, got your list? Now, once your eyes are closed, try to visualize each of those moments floating in its own balloon. You might have one or two balloons, or it might look like a balloon drop at Madison Square Garden. Imagine popping each of those balloons one by one and watching the contents return to the universe. They are not serving you, and you can return them to their owners now. Okay, *now* you can close your eyes. I'll see you back here in a few minutes.

TRAUMATIC GRIEF

Deaths that are violent, sudden, or accidental, losses witnessed firsthand, and those that occur prematurely (as is often the case for siblings) are all common examples of a traumatic loss—and they are—but that's not the whole story. As grief and trauma expert Gina Moffa explains, "A loss doesn't have to be traumatic to be traumatizing. See, loss of any kind is a shock to the system. It makes us question what we know to be true about ourselves, our place in the world, and so many of the things that we take (or took) for granted. For some people, loss isn't just life-altering; it's life-altering in a way that changes the way our minds and bodies feel safe in the world."[8]

If you had asked me in the first few years after Ben's death if I had experienced trauma, I would've said no. I would have told you that those men who were with him that day in Afghanistan and witnessed his death were traumatized. I would have told you that people whose lives and losses involved abuse or neglect, those who witnessed the death of their siblings, those who found their siblings' lifeless bodies—those people experience trauma. I hadn't read a single thing about trauma or traumatic loss, but I still managed to convince myself that what I had experienced didn't rise to the level of true trauma. Those other situations, those other siblings—they all had it worse than I did. They experienced real trauma; I had remained sheltered.

But I hadn't remained sheltered, not at all. My relationship with Ben was a textbook example of a secure attachment. To lose someone of that magnitude would be traumatizing for anyone because trauma is something that so completely overwhelms our nervous system it renders us unable to cope. Our brains and bodies switch into survival mode, and we go into fight or flight. It is the same response we experience when our own lives are threatened. I wonder if that is why so many siblings told me that they were convinced they, too, would die shortly after the death of their siblings.

When I finally did read about trauma and traumatic loss, I kept reading and rereading these lists of symptoms, and I could imagine big green checkmarks appearing next to each one. By that point I knew the panic attacks and nightmares were clearly a result of Ben's death, but there were things in those lists that I hadn't even considered could be connected:

- ✓ heart palpitations
- ✓ hypervigilance
- ✓ memory loss
- ✓ emotional numbness
- ✓ feelings of guilt
- ✓ "an overwhelming sense of fear and dread"[9]

and the list goes on.

I felt a powerful realization and affirmation come over me: I *did* experience a trauma. I *am* allowed to be this overwhelmed; in fact, it is completely logical and, dare I say, "normal" to be this . . . traumatized.

I had experienced a trauma. Full stop. No qualifiers.

Perhaps you have already had this realization and understanding around your own traumatic loss, or perhaps (like me) you don't see your own loss as traumatic because there are other people who have been through worse. Trauma isn't a competition, and it exists on a spectrum. No matter what anyone else has endured, that doesn't diminish what you've been through. Someone always "has it worse," but that won't serve you at all. Plus, your nervous system does not understand nuance, so in the most practical sense that argument is unlikely to do us any good. Our siblings are supposed to be our longest relationships, and if they're gone and you're still here, then it means they left us too soon; that's going to be traumatic. If you've been questioning this, and if it feels helpful to you, take a moment to allow yourself to give weight and validation to the very real impact trauma has had on your life.

Simply acknowledging to myself that I experienced a traumatic loss has been somewhat revolutionary. I've become nicer to myself, gentler. The trauma is still there, but at least I'm actively addressing it in therapy, and I'm no longer pretending it does not exist. I hope you can do the same for yourself—and I hope you can find someone to talk to who can reaffirm all of that for you. Trauma is real and it is serious, and left unaddressed it can lead to prolonged grief disorder. If you feel you're experiencing traumatic grief, or any kind of trauma, I encourage you to talk about it more deeply with a mental health professional. As a reminder, you can visit PsychologyToday.com, and on the top of the page you'll see "find a therapist"—look for someone in your area who specializes in grief and trauma.

DELAYED GRIEF

All the times we pretended to be fine and put others' grief before our own act as roadblocks on the path to healing. Healing, in this case, doesn't mean we stop grieving, but our grief changes shape, and if we experience complicated grief, it freezes our grief in its most acute and challenging form. Think of Cara, the older sister who didn't cry when her brother died because she went into caregiver mode and now seven years later reflected to me, "I thought I'd deal with it later, and I never did. Now my mom can talk about the loss all day, but I can't even say his name without crying."

Or the survey participant who shared that "I felt like I was not able to grieve as I was the person who had to be strong to make all the arrangements. Four years later and I'm sobbing as I am taking this survey because I have not had the opportunity to fully grieve." No matter the age or cause, delayed grief is just that—delayed. You cannot outrun it. You can grieve now or later (really, it's both), but you'll have to face it eventually. Grief runs a hell of a lot faster than you do. It's the Usain Bolt of emotions, and even if you get a twenty-year head start, it will, eventually, catch up to you.

Dorothy P. Holinger describes delayed or suppressed grief as "a sorrow that is not allowed its full expression."[10] Litigation or other extended processes related to a death can often lead to delayed grief, as the bereaved are overwhelmed by the trial, logistics, or media coverage, leaving them unable to focus on their grief. The deep grief may then erupt months or years later, triggered by a seemingly random event. Delayed grief and complicated grief may seem similar in that they are both prolonged, but I think of them as a slow cooker versus a pressure cooker. Complicated grief (the slow cooker) is grief that is apparent and remains simmering for extended periods of time. Delayed grief can cook an entire roast in fifty minutes once it has reached pressure; but sometimes it takes a while for that pressure to slowly, silently, build.

A NOTE ON ADOLESCENCE

Loss of a sibling is not experienced the same way for all ages, just as it is not experienced the same way for one individual throughout their lives. Losing a sibling in childhood and adolescence is distinctly different than in your thirties and beyond—which is why many therapists and grief counselors recommend people reprocess loss in their thirties.

So let's go back.

Studies have shown that loss in mid-adolescence "profoundly interrupts the progressive movement along a developmental path."[11] That's why one grieving sibling asked me if I'd found anyone else who felt like they're still frozen at the age they were when their sibling died.

After losing her brother junior year of high school, one sibling explained that while time stopped for her, it seemed to move at hyper speed in the world around her. "I went from being a star student to skipping classes to cry on the floor of my principal's office. My friendships deteriorated; what sixteen-year-old is equipped to support a friend during grief? I felt immense loneliness, while also feeling crystal clear clarity. The things I cared about once, I didn't care about anymore. I could no longer enjoy the trivial things my friends enjoyed. College was suddenly off the table due to falling grades. I wasn't supported by anyone so I learned to cope and hold myself together so my mom could grieve, to support her and grieve in private. Eventually I made new friends who I told about my past, but without emotion. I expressed sadness but never showed it; I lost my ability to be vulnerable with others."

While logically it makes sense that a fifteen-year-old would process, and express, death differently than a forty-five-year-old, that nuance is often lost in the moment. One study found that adolescents may have an exceptionally difficult time because their grief is layered on top of the intense challenges happening in their development. In my own research, I heard this sentiment again and again from adults who had lost their sibling during adolescence. Looking back, they could understand that time in a new way.

Consider the sibling whose brother was murdered when she was in high school, his death and subsequent trial all over the local news in their small town. Looking back, she recounted,

> I felt so alone, and because our whole family was grieving and I was still young, I don't feel my grief was noticed as much. I struggled in school, I struggled with friends. It was hard for me to emotionally regulate. I started a new school the year of his murder trial, and that's how I became known to other students at my new school. Kids learned about my brother through this public trial. I was bullied because of the many losses my family had already experienced. I was bullied by kids saying that anyone who became close with me would die. So it took me a while to make friends at my new school, in a time when I really needed support.

Unfortunately, the fact that her grief wasn't noticed is extremely common. One study on surviving siblings found that parents were not aware of the depth of trauma their own surviving children expressed because while 95 percent of siblings reported six or more symptoms of PTSD, only 40 percent of parents observed those symptoms in their children.[12] This isn't necessarily the parents' fault, and it is often the result of siblings internalizing their grief and intentionally hiding it in an attempt to shield their parents from additional pain and anguish. It's also because that whole "kids are so resilient—they'll be fine!" theory really only goes so far.

Some bereaved siblings, especially those who experienced the loss in adolescence, delay their own grief—either intentionally or unintentionally. In some cases, the postponement of grief is the unintended consequence of adolescents trying to act "normal" and unemotional to maintain social connections. Driven by a desire to fit in with their peers, many will watch their parents grieve with an almost distant quality, allowing the loss to be something experienced by their parents alone.

In other cases, or in combination with fitting in, some adolescents push the grief deep down inside themselves. Frightened by the powerful emotions they feel within and see on their parents' faces, many repress their own grief because they know no other way to control and process these powerful emotions.[13]

Adolescents are looking for permission.

Permission to grieve.

Permission to not be okay.

Permission to talk about it.

Permission to not talk about it.

Breanne was sixteen when she discovered her brother incapacitated by suicide and proceeded to call 911 and perform CPR while waiting for the paramedics. She wanted to talk about it, but there was no one to talk about it with.

> It's not that I didn't want to not talk about it. I was very open to that. The problem is that I had no one to talk to. My mother had made it clear that we weren't supposed to talk about it with anyone because he died by suicide. I wasn't put in therapy; my school didn't have me talk to a counselor; no teacher came and said, "Let's talk about this."

Nobody, none of the adults wanted to talk about it. The only person who did want to talk about it was my mom, but not to help me process the trauma and loss. She was grieving as a mother and wanted me to support her grieving process. I recognized, even as a teenager, it was not my job to support her. So I didn't talk about it because the only person who I was allowed to talk about it to was the person who actually needed a whole different source of support, and wasn't supporting me.

Those who experienced sibling loss as a child or adolescent must return as an adult—armed with the knowledge, love, and care needed to re-parent that sad kid inside who misses their sibling and never truly got the opportunity to give weight to their grief.

INHIBITED GRIEF

Many I spoke to, myself included, believed that the best way to help their parents—perhaps the only way that was within their control—was to pretend they were okay. We can't make it better, but we can try not to make it any worse. Study after study has illuminated a pattern of bereaved siblings intentionally hiding their grief from their parents. This could be driven by the desire not to upset their parents and be a burden, the belief that their parents' grief is worse than their own, or—often—both.

Kat told me that losing her brother "felt like something that had happened to my mom. She lost a kid. I don't want to add the burden of another kid being sad." This dynamic didn't develop after death; it was the pattern for as long as Kat could remember. Her role in the family was to not be the difficult one. Eight years after her brother's death, Kat was able to express to me that "not grieving has to do with not being the problem child and adding to her [mother's] problems."

Kat still dreams that her brother's death never happened. Eight years have passed since he died by suicide, and she suspects she has never truly grieved:

I feel a distance from his death; when I think about it, I don't feel the immediate, deep sadness about him that I know is in there. I just keep it at arm's length and haven't just been sad about it. It's been eight years! When you ask me questions and I tell you what he means to me I start to cry. I know that it's there. But I think it really does feel secondary. I think in my mind, still to this day, as I'm saying these words about how I know it's important for me to grieve him as a brother . . . it still feels like something that happened to my mom.

For others, hiding their grief was unintentional. When we spoke, it had been over three years since Devin's brother Baron died of complications from ulcerative colitis and blood clots after spending 112 days in the hospital, many with Devin by his side. After the funeral, Devin and their mom spent a week packing up Baron's apartment.

One of the things that I've realized is that I was doing the same thing for my mom that I had just been doing for Baron in the ICU. I held her in a way that let her know she's okay. So every morning I said, "Mom, we're taking a walk. We're going outside, we're moving."

I'd get up with her, we're both wrecks, but we'd stretch and walk. And she would say "What are we going to do now?" So I would try to keep it light and deep at the same time. Recently I realized, oh, wow, I didn't even feel anything because I was so busy making sure my mom was okay, because it's fucking hard to lose your son and, like, now you're going through his shit. And, like, we had great moments, but I was pretty numb for a while.

The dual loss grieving siblings experience, coupled with unhealthy family dynamics and self-imposed expectations, sends many into this protection mode.

Must protect whatever is left.

Must be okay.

Must reapply Band-Aid to gaping wound and ignore the infection.

Must be okay.

Fine.

It's fine.

This hidden grief obviously doesn't actually help anyone. If we aren't honest with our loved ones, how can we expect them to know what is really going on? It kicks off a painful cycle that can trap us for years.

Logic dictates that siblings would grieve. But logic doesn't play a role in grief. Grief is explicit. It's literal. There's no room for nuance, no shades of gray, no energy to excavate another person's emotions. So yes—people (parents, family, friends) may treat us like we aren't grieving—but feeding into that narrative and hiding our truth doesn't help anyone. It certainly won't help you. If we choose to hide our grief, it must also come with the understanding that we might do a really good job. We might remain hidden, and that's a prison of our own making.

QUIET GRIEF

There's an offshoot of inhibited grief that I'd like to propose: quiet grief. Grief that rips you apart on the inside but has no clear outlet. Grief that bounces around your mind and body. Grief that somehow remains invisible from the outside. This quiet grief is slightly different than inhibited grief. It's not a choice made to hide the truth in our grief; quiet grief is quiet by default. It is the grief desperate to get out but the host body (that could be you!) has nowhere else to put it.

Quiet grief is the grief of a sibling who only wants to talk about it with their brother or sister. For those of us with other surviving siblings, this quiet grief somehow isn't much easier. Chris has five surviving siblings, but it is hard to talk to any about it because none of them experienced the exact same version of their brother that he did—each had a slightly unique relationship with different memories and different struggles.

I often wonder why I didn't talk about it more with Sam in the early years. We spent time together, lived on the same street, and spoke nearly every day. I'm sure it was obvious to both of us that we were clinging to each other, but we didn't talk about it. The easy answer is that Ben was the brother I'd call to process emotions and dump my feelings. Sam was the brother I'd call to distract me from my feelings. Both were essential to me. Truth is, that answer would be a cop-out. I could have called Sam anytime day or night; I know that beyond a shadow of a doubt. I'd go to his apartment just to be near him and get that big brother hug, and perhaps I didn't need to go deep because it was unspoken. I didn't always talk about it with Sam because I was terrified he'd think *he* wasn't enough. That I loved Ben more. That I wasn't grateful every day for his mere existence. Is that logical? Once again, I truly do not care.

Quiet grief is also the grief of a sibling who doesn't have the vocabulary to mourn, in many cases because the cause of death is a taboo topic. Cara appeared visibly confused when I asked why she didn't talk about the loss with her family. "I'm not sure how we would . . . or why?" Sometimes it's not just the family's silence, but that of an entire community. It's Steven telling me, resigned, "We're Irish Catholic; we don't talk about feelings."

GRIEVING IN ISOLATION

Grieving is, historically, a team sport. No one on the team is good at the sport, the sport has no rules, and everyone hates playing it; but imagine it's a team sport. Football. I hate football, so let's make this a football analogy.

Grieving in isolation is like being trapped in an empty football stadium that's somehow both sweltering and freezing, and the only way out is to win. But you can't win because football is a team sport, and you're alone while the opposing team is stacked. You try to make a pass, but to whom? You try to run but you're tackled. And the cycle continues.

Okay, enough football—you get it.

Beginning in 2020, Covid-19 was the opposing team, and mourners were faced with an unprecedented level of isolation. It forced seclusion on those who would have found solace in community, a hug, the presence of another. One sibling who lost her brother to suicide early in the Covid-19 pandemic shared that "nothing about being prohibited to hug my parents or be surrounded by loved ones when I needed them the most felt natural or healing to me. I felt caged and alone and completely at a loss of how to regain a sense of self again."

About two years after my brother's death, I found myself in a windowless room in the Harvard Graduate School of Design watching my partner defend his dissertation. There were three students presenting that day, and I had planned to stay and support each one. The thesis presented after Aaron's was a new concept for cemeteries. He'd warned me of this, of course, but I thought it would be fine. LOL. While presenting her thesis, the student explained the layout and that, at times, mourners would walk single file. The space ebbed and flowed like breath, from open to narrow, narrow spaces. Unfortunately, my own breath became increasingly narrow, and I felt one of the panic attacks I'd become so familiar with taking hold.

You want me to walk to my brother's graveside . . . alone? You want me to follow his casket to its final resting place while staring at someone's back? You want my mother to walk alone, with no one beside her to hold her up? It was my nightmare. My breath picked up and people were looking at me. I tried to calm myself down, remind myself this was a theoretical design, it wasn't real. But the image of walking alone, with no one to hold my hand, was so deeply, deeply sad. Such a huge miscalculation of the human condition.

We were not meant to grieve in isolation.

SOMATIC SYMPTOMS

It has become a commonly accepted truth that stress is detrimental to our overall physical health. Yet when it comes to grief, many are blindsided by its physical manifestation. But what is grief if not the ultimate stressor? In grief, our cortisol levels (the stress hormone) are elevated and remain so for anywhere from six months to decades-plus. That factor alone comes with increased cardiac risk, decreased immune function, and an overall decrease in quality of life.[14] The shock and stress of grief can also overwhelm our brain's T cells, making us more susceptible to illness, and the increased cortisol leaves us vulnerable to both mental and physical illness in the future.[15]

Studies have shown that both social support and relationship type and strength positively correlate to the development of somatic symptoms, and unfortunately, siblings' disenfranchised grief and internalizing make for the perfect environment in which somatic symptoms can flourish. Somatic symptoms are so strong in siblings because when grief is repressed it still finds a way to manifest itself, except instead of tears or rage it comes in the form of headaches, insomnia, GI issues, nausea, or decreased sense of taste (seriously).[16] One sibling described it this way: "I wish people understood that sometimes this type of grief is physically debilitating. Sometimes having a shower is hard, let alone parenting my child or working my full-time job. Grief over losing my sibling has become another full-time job."

These somatic symptoms aren't on a schedule and can't be predicted. Just as cortisol levels may remain elevated chronically, so may the resulting physical manifestations. Treating each symptom is like playing a game of whack-a-mole. I guess some people find it fun (the game, not the symptoms), but I'd like a word with the masochist who invented that most frustrating, unwinnable game. The best way to "win" a game of whack-a-mole isn't to hammer at each individual mole but to address the root of the problem; unplug the damn machine and get some funnel cake with a friend. Seriously. Social support is, perhaps, the best treatment for these somatic symptoms that are essentially the manifestation of grief without a home or outlet. Now it's your job to find it another outlet, whether it be professional counseling or opening up to a friend (or both)—you need to find someone you can open up to, someone you can be honest with. Remember, grief always wins in the end.

Part II

Without

six

Parents Just Don't Understand

We're half-awake in a fake empire.

—The National

It's time to talk about our parents.

This chapter is hard to read and it was hard to write. I have two children and cannot fathom the pain my parents have experienced in the years since my brother's death. I don't know how they survived the funeral, the graveside burial, and each day that has passed since. What I *do* know is that they did their best. What follows is not an attack on parents, but a real, raw look at the impact loss can have on the family unit, and those who remain.

Interview after interview siblings expressed, with an almost resigned understanding, that their parents were not capable of being present during this time. Not that they didn't want to be present, but that they were incapacitated. In Sharae's family, she explained, parents cared for kids and the oldest kid (herself) cared for the younger ones. After her brother's death, her parents were despondent, and it was the first time she realized there was no one to take care of her—"there's no net here." Others described their parents as "nonfunctional," "distraught in a way I've never witnessed," and "despondent."

This dynamic is referred to as a dual loss because the bereaved sibling has lost both their sibling and the support of their parents.[1] It's a cruel twist of fate that when we need our parents the most, they are incapable of supporting us. As Sarah put it, after the loss of her brother, "I lost my parents too. They weren't emotionally present for years. Seeing your parents suffer is the ultimate pain." Kat described that her brother's death "permanently cracked my mom's mental health." Nearly every sibling told me they never see their parents smile the same way they used to.

The raw emotional grief displayed by parents can be disturbing to witness.[2] For younger mourners, in or barely out of adolescence, their grief and fear can be made worse through witnessing their parents' distress. They often see this distress as a manifestation of their own failure to be "enough" for their parents.[3]

Grieving parents are not ignorant of this shift, and yet they cannot control it. One study on complicated grief and PTSD noted that after losing a child, "parents can feel like they are losing their minds. Deep sorrow can be terrifying."[4] Therapists I've spoken with note that grieving parents know that they aren't showing up for their surviving children, often convinced they're not doing a "good job" supporting them, which in turn is a tremendous source of guilt and adds to their grief. While parents may feel guilty for not showing up, the truth is that they simply can't.

There's no solution here. No brilliant wise words. Losing a sibling *is* a dual loss. You *do* lose part of your parents. None of you will ever be the same.

A common thread in much of my research on the parental relationship is the acceptance and assumption that their parents did the best they could. Notably, some have only come to that after years of therapy and the benefit of hindsight. In the moment, and in the years of deep grief following their loss, bereaved siblings struggle to know how best to help and support their parents.

For some, their approach was to show that they were okay through their actions. The logic being, if my parents think I'm okay, they won't worry. If they don't worry about me, I'm not making their lives any harder. After Rob's sister died by suicide, he decided he was going to reassure his parents that things would be okay through his own actions.

> I can't reverse what's happened, so how do I move forward in a way that's going to create some sense of calm and joy and happiness in my immediate family? That became my focus. The better I could do at work, the better I could do with my personal relationships . . . all of these things that create life; your friendships, who I was dating, getting engaged, all these things. The better I could be at those, and the better news I could bring back to the family to distract, that was all I could do, and I'm happy to do it.

Others choose to actively care for their parents as a way of (consciously or unconsciously) avoiding their own grief. "I really did not cry when he died," Cara admitted. "I just went into caregiver mode and thought, 'I need to be there for my mom, I need to be there for my brothers, for my dad.' I thought I'd deal with this later, and then I just never dealt with it."

NO ROOM FOR OUR GRIEF

Just as we need to make space for imperfect siblings and the possibility that there are no good memories, we also need to acknowledge that there are imperfect parents—sometimes deeply so.

In some cases, the challenges that surrounded their sibling in life left little room for surviving siblings to have problems of their own. Time and time again, siblings shared the sentiment that there wasn't room for them to have big problems; they had to be the easy one, the strong one, the responsible one. This dynamic serves as a breeding ground for resentment within the family unit—both before and after a sibling's death.

In the immediate aftermath of the death, many bereaved siblings find themselves in a position they'd never imagined—planning the funeral and dealing with the logistics of laying their brothers and sisters to rest while also caring for their parents. This dynamic often leads to parentification, which may or may not have existed in the relationship previously. Parentification is a dynamic in which children in a family are pushed into more of a parent role than is developmentally appropriate.

The possible negative implications of parentification, especially in adolescence, cannot be understated. Many of the bereaved siblings who were put in this situation reported feelings of isolation, resentment, disenfranchisement, as well as delayed and/or complicated grief.

Rita felt she had to help everyone after her brother was shot, her mind racing with all the ways she needed to care for her other siblings and her mother while "this little voice in my head that even now still says, 'What about me? What about me?' Everyone was saying, 'You have to help your mother,' and I'm like, 'But what about me? Who is gonna help me?' I still feel like that now today. I don't talk to my mom or my siblings about how I feel because I'm so worried about how they feel." Ryan described it as the ultimate role reversal. "I'm still the kid," she recalled. "Does anyone care if I'm okay?"

Many of the grieving siblings I spoke to had been parentified long before their sibling's death. This added an additional layer of complexity in grief, as society focuses most on parental loss, and the parental role served by other surviving children is often ignored.

Molly was the only family member to visit her brother in jail. When he worked, she'd cash his checks for him, even though she knew he was using the money to buy heroin. She recounted the time when, at fourteen weeks pregnant, she was rushing from work to get his bail bond and tripped on the train platform and slid on her stomach. "I slid all the way to the edge of the tracks, like, to the bumps," she took a deep breath, "and I just thought why? Why is this happening to me? I'm doing all these things my parents just aren't around to do for him, and I started to feel this weight. I finally told him, 'Jason, I'm doing the best I can without Mom and Dad, I can't . . . I can't be everybody, somebody.'" After that she continued to bail him out because she didn't see any choice in the matter. "I needed to take care of Jason because our mom couldn't. She was incapable." But Molly *was* capable, so there she was—playing the role of mother to her peer, as resentment toward her own mother grew. The day her brother died, after being the one to tell her parents the news, Molly went back to her grandmother's house with her parents and other family members, and everyone started sharing their memories of her brother.

And I was very quiet looking at everybody, and they're like, "Oh, we're so grateful we had that lobster dinner with him four weeks ago." I asked, "What lobster dinner?" "Well, we all had this big dinner together . . . " and I said, "Why didn't you invite me?" "Well, we figured you were busy."

That's when I literally let loose on my family; all of this emotional baggage after years and years and years of having to care for and take care of all these precarious situations that are full of emotional baggage. It dawned on me . . . it's so great you guys all have this great fucking memory, but you never called me to make me part of it. Why? Why would you do that?

Some parents seemed to just . . . forget the sibling relationship entirely. That's something I don't understand, as both a parent and a sibling myself. When you have multiple children, there's so much focus on fostering a healthy relationship between them, but when one is gone, many parents seem to downplay the impact. I don't know if it's a coping mechanism or the pure selfishness of grief, but parents can forget their children mourn. Like Cara's mom, who, years after her son's death, commented that Cara "didn't seem to care" about her brother's death.

Cara responded simply, "You never asked."

PARENTAL OWNERSHIP

For better or worse, regardless of their track record, parents of the deceased are often the "owners" of not only grief, but the narrative, decisions, and physical belongings surrounding our lost siblings. In some cases, if the deceased was married, this role will fall to their spouse, but parents are still the narrators and arbiters of their children's lives—deciding what will happen to their belongings, what traditions are observed after death, and what does—and does not—get acknowledged.

For many of the siblings I spoke to who were impacted by physical or mental illness, including addiction, these dynamics began long before their sibling's death. Sarah had been terrified when her younger brother got into drugs in middle school, and as much as she tried to ring the alarm bells, her parents always reassured her that it would be fine. The worst word in the English language: "fine." That dismissal didn't bring her any actual comfort; it only served to fuel her fears because it was *not* fine, and it seemed like her parents weren't taking it seriously. Her fears were never validated. "I still remember where I was when I found out that he was using heroin. I was devastated. My parents kept it from me, they kept a lot of things from me." I asked how she'd found out. "I was sitting on the couch," she began, "and my dad said he'd taken my brother to the doctor. So I asked why, and he wouldn't answer, so I asked again . . . And then he said, 'Well, he has a little infection in his arm.'" That's when she knew it was heroin. No one had told her, but now they didn't have to.

Sarah blamed her parents for years after her brother's overdose. With time, she has come to accept that they did the best they could and were trying to protect her. Parents are often in an impossible situation. If they put too much on their surviving child (before or after the loss), they risk parentification. If they try to handle it all themselves, without involving their other kids, they run the risk of dismissing valid concerns and putting their child's trust in jeopardy. They cannot win. There is no easy way.

Throughout my interviews I observed an interesting split—those who took care of everything, and those who knew nothing.

After Jay's sister's traumatic brain injury, she lived at home with around-the-clock nursing care. As her health deteriorated, her immune system weakened, and eventually any cold or illness became dire for her. "She went to a school program every day," he explained, "and I remember that I did not kiss her goodbye the night before or in the morning before she left that day. My parents picked me up from school and told me she was gone. That was it. She had pneumonia and my parents said the doctors couldn't drain her lungs. I never got any other specific information beyond that." Imagine not even owning the information surrounding the death. Having a gatekeeper to the details of how your brother or sister died. In many cases, they can also be the gatekeeper to help, support, and community. As Jay put it,

> I was never allowed to grieve. My parents never got me any counseling or therapy, not even one meeting. It was never even mentioned. We got on with our lives. It was basically, "We're all sad and we miss her. But things like this happen and now she's in a better place." I didn't know how to feel, and I often felt nothing at all. There was no processing of feelings.

A 2017 study on sibling grief found that a common area of distress for bereaved siblings was in the treatment of their deceased sibling's belongings, including their childhood bedroom. One sister recounted her parents' decision to shut the door to her brother's room the day he died, and she was not allowed inside. She proceeded to write letters to her brother and would slide them under his closed door. Another remembered that the photos of her brother were taken off the wall the day after he died, and as a result, "it was like Robert never existed."[5] This dynamic was perfectly illustrated in Breanne's story. After her brother died by suicide in their apartment, Breanne explained,

> My mother didn't want to go back to where we were living. So she had friends pack up all of our stuff; I was never allowed back into our home. We moved in with my mom's boyfriend who lived thirty minutes away from everyone and everything, my school. All my stuff was put in boxes, and I was sent to this place where nobody knew where I was, right? Like, I was a teenager and none of my friends or the people in my life knew where

I was. I was just kind of sent away. I had none of my belongings, or my brother . . . it wasn't just one thing; all the things were stripped away at once. Everything was removed from my life all at once.

FAMILY DYNAMICS

When you lose a sibling, your entire family life and reality can be thrown off-kilter. You're left grieving not only the individual who is gone, but your entire family unit. Rob described it as a "nuclear bomb detonating in our home. Nothing was recognizable again."

That description is, unfortunately, extremely accurate. Study after study has shown that the loss of a child (whether in childhood, adolescence, or adulthood) throws the family into crisis and disrupts any balance that may have existed. A family is a structure built of individual bricks; if a single brick is removed, the entire structure changes. Sometimes with a dramatic collapse, other times a gaping hole or a wobbly foundation, constantly threatening collapse. This shift in dynamics can be delayed. The family structure may appear stable, only to deteriorate years later. Or it can also work in reverse—a family working together to rebuild the structure with the remaining bricks while acknowledging their loss.

In either scenario, there's a deep level of grief directed at the family unit itself. Whether you come through the loss closer or forever fractured, it will be different from the family dynamic you're used to—and different from any family you likely imagined. It's okay to mourn the family that once was, with all its imperfections and dysfunctions. That was your family, it was the only family you've ever known, and now that family is no more.

I never fantasized much about my wedding, but there were a few elements that I'd assumed were a given. I would wear a really pretty dress, my dad would walk me down the aisle, and my brothers would walk my mom down the aisle before finding their place under the chuppah with me. Wedding planning after Ben died was more emotionally complex than I could have predicted. We ended up planning a destination wedding as an excuse to keep it very (very) small, and we did not have a wedding party. I couldn't do it. I could not have a wedding party that didn't include both brothers. In the months leading up to my wedding, my family attended the wedding of Sam's best friend. The three kids in Michael's family lined up perfectly with our own, and we'd all gone to school together since kindergarten. We were mirrors of each other; or at least we had been. As Michael's brother and sister stood up to give a toast, I noticed my mom quietly slipping away from the party and walking down toward the water. I followed her, concerned that this was all too much and she was upset. As I'd feared, she was crying when I found her, but she surprised me by pulling me in close and whispering, "I'm sorry, I'm so sorry," over and over in my ear.

"Why are you sorry?" I asked, confused. "No one else noticed you're gone. It's fine!"

"No, Annie, I'm sorry. I'm sorry to you."

I wasn't following and asked, "Mom, what could you possibly be sorry for?"

"You're supposed to have both your siblings at your wedding. They're both supposed to be there to give a toast. I'm sorry I couldn't keep him safe; that was my job and I couldn't do it."

My heart broke in that moment, and here I am crying as I recount it eleven years later. I wasn't the only one who had lost that image of my future. My mother had also imagined my wedding; she'd also imagined walking down the aisle flanked by her towering boys; she'd envisioned all three kids standing beside one another at this (and every) milestone event. We were all mourning the family we'd had for so long.

THE NEW OLDEST

Most siblings I spoke with expressed that within this new family dynamic they've been forced to assume a new role. In addition to the pressure of caring for parents and family members while facing our own grief, there are shifting dynamics at play that redefine our place in the family unit. Birth order is a conflicting topic, but there is no denying the fact that birth order does shape us in many ways.

Externally, consider how many times judgments or assumptions about your character have been made based solely on your birth order—the responsible oldest child, the ignored middle problem child, the spoiled baby, the selfish only child. But what happens when the middle becomes the oldest? The oldest or youngest becomes the only?

This is one transition that I didn't need to wrestle with personally. I'd been the baby, and I remained the baby. As was my way, being the baby and all, I called my big brother and asked if he'd felt the shift. "Oh, yeah!" he exclaimed before I'd even gotten the full question out.

"Remember, I gave his eulogy, that's why. There was all kinds of things I had to do because I was the oldest now, things Ben would have done if he was here."

"Why did you have to do it? You mean Mom and Dad asked you to?"

He paused, clearly thinking on the other end of the line. "No, no one asked. I guess I just knew it's what I had to do. I sat in the front seat." I wasn't sure what he meant at first, but he quickly continued, "With Major Dan, that day, I sat in the front seat. I wanted Mom and Dad to sit together; someone needed to sit in the front seat, so I sat in the front. It was a lot of things like that." He was referring to the drive from my parents' home in New Haven, Connecticut, to Dover Air Force Base in Delaware, driven by our bereavement officer who held our hands through those first few weeks and whom we lovingly called Major Dan (because he was a major and his name really was Dan, how great is that?). That was the ride I chose not to take; instead, I volunteered to tell my grandma the news because it seemed more palatable than taking the long drive to see Ben's body transferred from one military plane to another. But Sam went. He went and he sat in the front seat. A firstborn reporting for duty.

"I felt that for the first few years, but at some point . . . I don't know. Now I'm 1,000 percent back to being the middle child. I'd say I'm very, very much the middle child again. But in the beginning, yeah, I did feel like I needed to step up. No one asked me to. I just knew I needed to do it."

I think his return to feeling like a middle child is the perfect embodiment of resilient grief. He was able to take on whatever role needed to be filled at the time, but he did not let it redefine his identity. He didn't linger in it. Instead, he let the experience stretch and grow everything he was capable of, and he somehow found himself again in the process.

Chris was more explicitly expected to "step up" and resume the role his oldest brother had occupied in the family, and so far nothing about that has changed. His parents refer to him as "the new Tom" and tell him, "Your job is to take care of your siblings, like Tom did." But Chris isn't Tom, and the family he's working with is not the same family that existed when his brother was alive. This has led to a feeling of failure, as he told me, "I'm obviously doing a terrible job at it"—but that's not true at all! He's doing everything he possibly can; there is no going back, and that expectation is unrealistic. It's a fantasy.

THE NEW ONLY

Siblings who found themselves forced to operate as only children expressed different struggles. Many felt they had a bright spotlight on them, expected to live for both themselves and their sibling, and that attention wasn't comforting; it was suffocating. "It is really overwhelming," one sister told me, "because I don't want all this like attention on me. I don't need my parents to rectify any mistake they made with my brother through me. I don't want it." In addition to remedying mistakes, some siblings report that their parents put extra pressure on them to be successful, happy, or otherwise "okay" because—as the only child—the future seems to rest on their shoulders alone.

Being left as the only child also means that as their parents age, they're left to help and support them on their own. Of course, there are plenty of only children who are put in this position, but the dynamic is different for those who always expected to have a peer by their side. One bereaved sister noted that dealing with her aging parents is now "an unexpected, recurring reminder of my loss."

ASSUMING GRIEF

In addition to hiding their own grief, many siblings find themselves taking on the grief of others, adding even more weight to the invisible burden they carry. Most often, the grief they took on was that of their parents—making themselves available night and day, troubleshooting, listening, comforting. It sounds lovely, right? What a good kid to be there for their parents like that.

But it's not good, not for the child at least—not without some boundaries.

When we put other people's grief before our own, we set ourselves up for delayed, complex grief. The result? We wake up one day and realize our parents are okay. Everyone else is okay, but we're not. For us, the journey is just beginning and it can be impossible to catch up.

Caring for, and owning, the emotions of their parents was so prevalent in my interviews that when I spoke to someone who *hadn't* fallen into that pattern, I'd always try to understand . . . how?

Kim told me she'd been overwhelmed by the calls from her mother asking her to help troubleshoot her loss. "What did you do?" I asked. Kim took a breath and said, "I lovingly told her I'm trying to have a good day, and I can't take on your grief right now."

Sometimes the most powerful responses are the simplest.

I can't take on your grief right now.

It's essential that we work on our own grief and not the grief of others. It's easy to focus on your parents—for some of us it feels impossible not to—but they can get through their grief just like you can. They're adults. You do not own their pain.

seven

Everything Doesn't Happen for a Reason

I know there's always something we have to go through / That has some deeper meaning but / Right now I just can't say / I know there's gonna be a lesson somewhere / I'm gonna think a lot about it later / Right now I'm miles away.

—Marc Cohn

People tell you lies when you're mourning. They're not lying intentionally (at least not *all* of them); they don't know what to say, so they say what they were taught. Unfortunately, most of us were taught lies.

When you lose a sibling, there can be a large delta between what people say and what you hear.

What They Say	**What We Hear**
Everything happens for a reason.	It's for the best.
They're in a better place.	Being dead is better than being here with you.
They would have wanted you to _____	I knew them and their wants better than you, so let me explain them to you.
I just heard your sibling died—I'm so sorry! How are your parents? They must be devastated.	I care enough to ask about your parents but not about you. I assume you're doing fine.
You two weren't close, were you?	You shouldn't be so upset.
I remember when my grandpa died . . .	Losing a sibling is like losing an elderly grandparent.

This type of response, dismissal of the mere possibility that you're grieving, is a form of disenfranchised loss (check out Chapter 5 for a refresher). It is also, unfortunately, how many people have been taught to deliver condolences. As if putting a positive spin on the loss will actually make someone feel better about it. We have been taught to say things like "they're not suffering anymore" when someone dies after an extended illness, as if the bereaved will hear our words and think, "Wow, I never thought of it that way! You're right, they're not suffering anymore so this is all totally okay!" We've been taught lies. Trying to find the silver lining in someone's loss doesn't heal their pain. After you've gotten a few of these zingers for the third, fourth, fifth, or seventy-eighth time, it's understandable that you might stop talking to people about your loss. After all, repeating the same thing and expecting a different response is lunacy, isn't it?

The unpredictability in how others respond to our grief, coupled with the likeliness that their response will make us feel worse, rather than better, further drives the urge to conceal grief. Siblings told me how they'd tried to keep track of who knows and who doesn't know, so they know if/when they need to prepare themselves for a new reaction. The question of "how many siblings do you have?" was universally dreaded among the bereaved siblings I spoke to, as many of them felt anxious about how they'd respond and fixated on their possible answers when meeting new people.

The first time I was faced with the question, I was in an S&M dungeon in Manhattan with Jason Schwartzman. It'd be funnier to leave it at that, but I'll explain. My brother Sam was a writer on the HBO series *Bored to Death*, and in the months following Ben's death, Sam would often call me from filming locations around the city and invite me to set. That day, they were filming two blocks from my school, and I eagerly raced over on a break between classes. Standing there, below a ceiling of whips and handcuffs, Jason Schwartzman casually turned to Sam and me and asked, "So, do you have any other siblings?" I froze. I could not speak and looked at him like I couldn't understand the question. I could not find the words, perhaps because I didn't actually know the answer. Did we? Do we? Is it only us now?

Losing a sibling requires us to learn a new language. In grief one becomes a widow, not a wife; an orphan, not a daughter; but there is no name for us. And then there are the tenses. Those loathsome tenses.

"Ben *is* thirty-two" became "Ben *was* thirty-two."

"You two *will* get along so well" became "You two *would have* gotten along so well."

"Ben *is* the first person I'd call with a problem" became "Ben *was* the first person I'd call with a problem."

"We *have* an older brother" became "We *had* an older brother."

Unless you're significantly older than your sibling, you might not remember a world in which there was no future tense. Sure, I could refer to Ben in the past tense when he was alive, recounting stories or speaking of missed opportunities. But now the past tense was all I had. Ben, as a person, was in the past.

That day in the S&M dungeon, Sam answered Jason when I could not, and you know what? I'm not going to tell you what he said. Because here's the truth: you can answer that question any way you want. In fact, you don't even have to answer it consistently! I've tried out a lot of different answers these past twelve years, and I have yet to find a one-size-fits-all response. Typically, I say that I *have* two brothers, because I've found that saying, "I have one brother" or "I had two brothers" makes me sad. For me, the joy in acknowledging that I still have him—that I still have two brothers—outweighs any sadness that could be triggered by follow-up questions. Then there are times when I answer that I have one brother because I simply do not want to get into it with whoever is asking. It's not a reflection of how much I love Ben, but an understanding that I own this information and I can share it when, where, and with whom I see fit. I do not owe anyone my story and neither do you.

A NEW VOCABULARY

Learning this new language while dealing with unwanted comments and misguided overtures is exhausting. Luckily, you quickly learn that if you don't talk to anyone, you don't need to learn the language. Easy peasy! Problem solved! It's no wonder, then, that so many report experiencing an element of social isolation after the death of their sibling. This isolation could be self-imposed or external, or both.

In my experience, if you're twenty-five years old and lose your brother in a violent, traumatic way, it's difficult for your friends to relate. Sure, a few of my friends had experienced loss—some had lost a parent, many had lost grandparents, but no one had experienced anything like this. I don't blame them for not knowing what to do, they had no example to follow, but I lost a lot of friends in the year after Ben died. This sense of isolation, alienation, and disconnection is all too common among grieving siblings.

The first time I went to the movie theater after Ben died, we went to see Spike Jonze's *Where the Wild Things Are*. It seemed like a safe bet— what could possibly be triggering about a story I practically know by heart? Well, when Max first meets the Wild Things, he tells them that he once became king of another land by making their heads explode. This, in turn, led to a discussion about whether Max could make the Wild

Things' heads explode, how he explodes heads, and how big everyone's heads are. For most people the scene is an endearing, childlike exchange, but not for someone whose brother's head had exploded a few months earlier. That was when I had my first panic attack, right there in the movie theater. After that, I wouldn't go see anything that I thought could be remotely triggering. That included the year's anticipated blockbuster, *Avatar*. I remember telling my friends I didn't want to see it because it involved war and got the same response over and over: "They're blue creatures, they're not even human." What I heard was, "Stop being dramatic" or "We're sick of your grief." So I stopped. I stopped trying to go out, trying to relate, trying to explain. How could anyone possibly understand anyway?

In exploring the social repercussions of sibling loss, one study found that "a sense of isolation and alienation from others was common for a time period after the death, especially in cases of intense media coverage or when people gossiped about the death. . . . Participants reported a feeling of being disconnected from people who may say the wrong thing, try to make the sibling happy, or tire of dealing with the grief."[1] Social isolation and alienation in grief are not without their repercussions. One follow-up study on young adults two to nine years after losing a sibling to cancer showed that the majority had not worked through their grief, and a small group had not worked through their grief *at all.* The factors most associated with not working through grief? Lack of social support and more recent loss.[2]

CAUSE OF DEATH

The type and amount of support surviving siblings receive are often determined (perhaps subconsciously) by the cause of death. In my research, cause of death was the single biggest predictor of the social response—more than relationship strength, birth order, or age. I imagine that all the lies people tell you when you're grieving come from the same book, with prompts and instructions to determine the "correct" response. This book contains chapters like

1. "They didn't feel any pain; and other things you can say after a violent death."
2. "Does suicide make you uncomfortable? Ignore it!"
3. "They were sick and now they're not; and other ways to make death sound like a vacation."
4. "Addiction isn't real and mental health is NBD; ten easy ways to blame the victim."

Alas, these categories are not as discrete as they seem since life and death are rarely cut-and-dry. The violent death of someone with a history of addiction; the suicide of someone suffering from chronic illness, trauma, or both; illness after years of unrelated (or related) substance abuse. People like a clean explanation. A nicely labeled bucket to put each of our emotions in. Problem is, that's not how life works, and you will likely find elements of your experience in each of the scenarios below because we are all a multitude of different things, and that's okay. You and your emotions don't need to fit into someone else's categorization.

SUICIDE

The aftermath and grief of losing someone to suicide is (as we've established) very different than the loss I'd experienced. During our interview, Rob patiently attempted to explain the conflicting feelings he experienced after his sister died by suicide. "It's a death that is endlessly unclean. It's, it's . . ." he paused. "It's got jagged edges and there's very little that you can do to smooth those out."

Suicide's jagged edges are all the points where you try to hold on tight—to control the reality unfolding in front of you—but you can't. This is not something within your control. After Stephen's brother died by suicide, he reflected, "It wasn't an overdose and that's almost more depressing. We got the toxicology report back and there was nothing in his system, he did this totally of sound mind. He thought this out, and that is almost more depressing to realize he had this whole thing planned."

In lieu of control, many siblings I spoke to sought answers.

Why did this happen?

What does this say about my sibling?

Did they not love us enough?

Did they not know how much we loved them?

Could I have done something to prevent it?

Questions of "what if?" abound among siblings grieving a suicide. But just as you, dear reader, do not possess the power to cure cancer or prevent war, you also do not possess the ability to alter someone's mental health or cure their addiction.

All of those questions are centered on us, the survivors. It's not about us. One layer deeper lie the questions about *them*, questions that can be much more frightening.

How much pain must they have been in?

How did they make this decision?

Did they know they were loved?

While those questions are not easy, they are essential. Acknowledging the depth of pain and despair their siblings must have felt may put their actions into stark relief. For some grieving siblings, this allowed them to find some peace, knowing how much they must have wanted the pain to stop.

Rather than being comforted, these siblings find themselves comforting others when the topic of suicide comes up. Chris described the shift that happened after his brother's suicide—the times he found himself trying to make the other person in the conversation feel better about having brought it up. As a result, he felt like he'd never had the opportunity to truly have the conversations that could have been most helpful. "You don't get a chance to have conversations about something like sibling loss; no one ever says, 'Man, it must really suck to lose your older brother who was your safety net in life,' and you can just say, 'Shit, it really was. It was awful. It was terrible.' And you just don't get to do it, not with suicide."

There's a morbid curiosity surrounding both suicide and violent death, and people feel comfortable asking questions of siblings that they wouldn't dare ask a parent. Let's take the classic: "How did they do it?" or "How did it happen?" Maybe it's the result of too many *True*

Crime podcasts or *Dateline* episodes, but some people feel entitled to the intimate details surrounding death without much concern for how the deceased lived, or how you are trying to survive. Those people who ask for the most from us are often the ones who give the least. Those who we trust know we'll share when we're ready, but those who ask don't want to wait.

You don't need to answer any question you aren't 100 percent comfortable answering. Let's practice.

[upon learning of your sibling's death by suicide]

Scenario 1:
    Them: That's terrible, I'm so sorry! How did they do it?
    You: I'd rather not go into details.

Scenario 2:
    Them: That's terrible, I'm so sorry! How did they do it?
    You: I don't want to discuss it right now.

Scenario 3:
    Them: That's terrible, I'm so sorry! How did they do it?
    You: [LITERALLY ANYTHING.]

ADDICTION

The grief of addiction often begins long before (technical) death, and many siblings report at least some anticipatory grief in the months or years preceding death. As Sarah explained, "The thing about substance abuse is that you have to grieve when they're alive, a lot. The first missed holiday is not when they died. The first time you think about them dying is not when you heard that they died. The loss of the relationship is not when they died." Because so much grieving has taken place before the physical death, siblings may be surprised when their own grief doesn't look like they'd expected. The grief they'd been wrestling with since learning of the addiction was now mixed with relief. A relief some were ashamed to voice out of fear that it would diminish their own loss. After all, these siblings wanted to see an end to addiction, not an end to life. If you experienced this relief, I need you to understand that it is completely normal and is not a reflection of your love for your sibling.

After Kim's brother died, she admitted, "One of the things that I had felt a lot of shame about was the relief. That's something I should tell you. I felt a lot of relief when he died and that brought me a lot of troubling feelings. Our relationship had felt really burdensome; I was constantly having crises come up, and my husband and I would talk about what we're going to do when Zach is fifty years old and wants to crash with us because he can't keep a home. We were always thinking about this. I did experience a sense of relief, which feels really awful because people who die by suicide feel like a burden. It is really hard to both acknowledge that there were burdensome feelings, and also I wouldn't have wanted him to die, ever."

Your relief is not a reflection of your love.

Once more in all caps so you know I'm yelling: YOUR RELIEF IS NOT A REFLECTION OF YOUR LOVE.

Feeling relieved doesn't mean you're not devastated.

This grief/relief combo is often accompanied by guilt that sits like a weight on your chest. That guilt is most often fueled by external forces. Those quiet (or loud) people telling you how you should be grieving— what you should feel. And so if you don't feel those things—or if you feel them but you feel more than that—the default assumption can be to blame yourself.

"I didn't know how to grieve," Juliet told me of the eight years follow- ing her brother's death from alcoholism. "Why didn't I grieve? Why was I okay?" At this point in our conversation, Juliet had told me how she'd mourned her brother's lost potential when they were young adults, and that she thinks about how much his addiction had influenced their entire family. So I offered to be the mirror to her grief—not just the grief that accompanied death but also the grief that swelled throughout his life. I asked if, perhaps, she knew his death was an inevitability and had already spent much of her life grieving. There was a moment of silence before she said, "That hits the nail on the head of something I could never figure out, which is, why didn't I grieve in the same way? And the reality is, I was already grieving for years, and I never thought of that. That's like, better than anything my therapist ever said to me." She laughed, as if in disbelief. "Oh . . . my . . . yeah, that's a very powerful statement. Yeah . . . I was already grieving him."

As with anything in life, we must understand that two (seemingly) conflicting emotions can reside within us at the same time. Grief and optimism, relief and devastation, fear and release.

As Juliet went on, I admired how she was able to hold her loss and relief in balance without the guilt-fueled, negative self-talk. "It sounds horrible, but I did feel that sense of relief and I wasn't guilty. I was sad for what I lost; I lost my sibling, but I did not feel guilty for being relieved."

Feel what you feel. Allow yourself to feel it without guilt or shame and own those emotions. Denying them will only carve them deeper into your psyche.

ILLNESS

Depending on the type of illness, many siblings report grief beginning months (or years) before the death, often ramping up in the late stages of the illness during which time some became their sibling's primary caretaker.

Sarah quit her job and moved in with her sister, spending weeks at a time in the hospital. Devin would leave his home in LA for weeks at a time to be at his brother's bedside in NYC, returning home only when he needed to take a job that would carry him through his next trip. Julie and Sarah both lost their sisters to genetic disease—one they were spared from despite carrying the same genes. A game of Russian roulette.

After their siblings passed, many were encouraged (or pressured) into returning to their old lives and routines. As if watching their siblings suffer was a detour rather than a fork in the road.

"Now you can get back to your own life."

"You must be relieved."

Yes, you might feel relief. You might find tremendous relief knowing they're no longer in pain. But that's up to you. No one else has the right to make that demand of you. Because regardless of intentions, those platitudes only further the internal critic who tells you you're doing it all wrong. You aren't doing it wrong.

VIOLENT OR ACCIDENTAL DEATH

The response to violent or accidental death can be strikingly similar to suicide and illness in some ways, and utterly unique in others.

When faced with violent or accidental death, society is both deeply unsettled and extremely curious. The topic can make others uncomfortable, driving surviving siblings to downplay or hide their sibling's cause of death so as not to upset others. Claudia told me that after her brother was murdered, she learned to talk in euphemisms to make other people feel better. "I don't say my brother was murdered," she told me. "That's very, very harsh language. What I've realized is that I change how I speak about it depending on who I'm talking to because I want to take their feelings into account. But then I'm the one who had to deal with this shit; do I really need to make my trainer at the gym, like, feel okay about this?"

One sibling recounted that because her brother's murder was drug-related, people tried to justify it. Everyone from the defense attorney at his trial to close friends and even family. Some may find themselves rushing to defend their siblings, making sure it's clear that their sibling was a good person. Rita remembers "making sure people knew he didn't get killed because he was involved in a gang. When you say he was killed they might ask if it was an accident, but when I say he was shot they're like, 'What did he do?' You know what, he died and it doesn't matter how. He died and we lost him and that's really all that matters."

Perhaps driven by a need to understand their own mortality and chance, when violent or accidental death is involved, some will want to know all the details. As if them knowing could prevent their own loved ones from meeting the same fate. As if the details may help them determine "fault" and how much sympathy you're due.

Were they the victim or the perpetrator?

Was this a sudden accident or did they see it coming?

Here's an example of how the conversation often goes when I share my own loss with new people:

Them: Can I ask . . . how did he die?

Me: He was killed in Afghanistan.

Them: Oh my god, that's terrible! I'm so sorry!

Them (quieter): What . . . what happened?

Me: He was killed by a suicide bomber.

Them: I'm so sorry.

Them (much quieter): Oh, I'm so sorry. Was he killed immediately? I hope?

This could go on and on, depending on just how curious the other person is. I know I could end the conversation, but the truth is, sometimes I enjoy answering those questions. It gives me a reason to talk about him, to share his story so that one more person can carry his legacy. Of course, I'd rather be talking about his life, but sometimes it's better than not talking about him at all. Talking about the details can be incredibly cathartic, and it is essential that each of us find someone we trust to unpack those details with. We need to tell the story—our story and theirs—to make any sense of it. The important thing to remember is that you own that conversation. You decide who gets to know the details. You decide who knows your story. You decide when, where, how, and with whom it is shared.

You don't need to speak in euphemism—but if it feels right to you, in that moment, then you should.

You don't need to reveal any details; you owe nothing to anyone—but if it feels good to talk and recount the events, then do it.

You own this story. Your story. And you get to select the audience.

eight

Anger, or Practical Uses for Ikea Dishes

For many men there is so much grief / and my mind is proud
but it aches with rage / and if I live too long I'm afraid I'll die /
strangers on this road we're on / we are not two, we are one.

—The Kinks

To grieve is to ride an uncontrollable rollercoaster that would never pass even the most basic safety inspection. A rollercoaster that can ricochet your body and mind from sadness to exhaustion to all-consuming rage without warning. It's often the rage that comes as the greatest surprise. It certainly was for me. The year Ben died, the Avett Brothers came out with a song called "Head Full of Doubt"; it's one of the songs that played on a loop while I rode the rage-coaster, the words "there's a darkness inside me that's flooded in light" resonating more and more each time I heard them.

The darkness inside me was the rage, and to have that darkness flooded in light is something I didn't anticipate. It's the moment the rage boils over. Shortly after Ben died, after yet another man had told me to "smile" while I'd been crying silently on the 6 train, I felt it. As I got off the train, rage grew inside me and I felt possessed. I needed to break something, I needed to punch and kick and throw. I needed to cause destruction. The feeling frightened me. I'm not an aggressive person, not by a long shot, and I had never felt this out of control with rage before. As I entered my apartment, I began to scan my belongings, as if through new eyes—these things didn't matter, they were just that, things. Nearly everything in this apartment was replaceable; none of it mattered at all. I could break whatever I wanted and it wouldn't matter. None of it would bring my brother back, and none of it could ever replace him.

I picked up a stack of Ikea plates, walked to the building's garbage chute, and threw the first plate inside like a frisbee. It smashed on the back wall, and I could hear the pieces break again as they collected at the bottom of the chute.

That felt good.

I did it again. And again. And again. Throwing the plates in with all my might, just to hear them shatter and fall into the abyss.

When I was finished, I walked slowly back into the apartment and collapsed on the couch, impressed with myself that all the plates actually landed in the chute and not all over the hall. Then the sudden realization that the maintenance staff was going to find, and have to clean, a mess of shattered plates struck me down with so much guilt that I started sobbing. I hadn't gotten my pain out—I'd transferred it. I'd made someone else's life harder just to spare myself a moment of anger. Someone was going to have to clean up my mess. The mess I'd made in the garbage chute as if it were a black hole that would take my anger away forever, but it wasn't a black hole. Nothing was going to magically erase this pain. My relief was replaced with wracking guilt and regret. What was I going to do now? Staring down the barrel of another night at home, alone, drowning in sadness and fear, and now guilt on top of it all.

Interview after interview, siblings told me about the anger—the darkness—inside them that was flooded with light for the first time. Anger they couldn't control and that, at times, frightened them.

But that's just it—it was an admission I heard over and over and over because no one told us to expect it or that it was okay to feel it. The anger shouldn't be a secret, and it doesn't need to be a surprise. The anger is normal. The anger is feeling. Processing. Realizing.

THE SHOCK OF ANGER

Studies on children and adolescents suffering the loss of a sibling have shown the prevalence and impact of this anger, noting not only its existence but that siblings were surprised by their unprovoked anger that would erupt in response to routine interactions.[1] Siblings in my survey expressed the same, many noting that they're now quick to trigger. They find themselves getting upset and angry unexpectedly and struggle to control it.

This can manifest in different ways depending on your life stage and unique situation. In childhood, studies have shown that bereaved siblings show increased behavioral issues[2] and elevated instances of aggressive behavior—along with a variable grab bag of challenges including depression, social withdrawal, and eating disorders.[3]

Have you ever read *The Catcher in the Rye*? I read it in middle school English class, as many of us were told to do. Over twenty-five years later, I remembered it as a book about an asshole kid in boarding school who called everyone a phony—and that's it. That's what I remembered. I don't remember Holden's grief ever being a topic of discussion in that class or in anything I'd heard about the book since. Holden's grief is everything. You see, *The Catcher in the Rye* is a story of sibling grief. It is the story of a sixteen-year-old boy who, at thirteen, lost his beloved brother Allie to cancer and has been getting himself kicked out of boarding school ever since in an attempt to go back home. It's a story of the anger, social withdrawal, aggression, and behavioral issues that are hallmarks of adolescent sibling grief. Early on in the book, Holden references his injured hand—the hand he reveals was broken the night Allie died when he used it to break all the windows in their garage: "It was a very stupid thing to do, I'll admit, but I hardly didn't even know I was doing it, and you didn't know Allie." That broken hand landed him in the hospital, forcing him to miss Allie's funeral—alone and isolated while the rest of his family grieved and experienced that first moment of closure.

My Ikea dishes were Holden's garage windows.

Holden was like many of the siblings I spoke with, struggling to channel the anger. He so desperately wanted someone to blame—someone he could direct that anger toward.

GIVING THE FINGER TO EVERYONE

Like many parts of grief, anger is an expert shape-shifter, taking different forms for different people and often assuming multiple forms at different stages of our lives. The anger is a firehose whose target keeps changing. Anger is the famous scene from *Half Baked*, a disgruntled employee shouting, "Fuck you!" at his coworkers.

Fuck you, parents.

Fuck you, siblings.

Fuck you, murder.

Fuck you, society.

Fuck you, pharmaceutical industry.

Fuck you, universe.

The anger isn't necessarily immediate; that's how it really gets you. The anger creeps up on you. "As time has gone on," one sibling reflected, "I've started to experience more anger surrounding the loss of my sister. Angry each time I see the devastation on my parents' faces, angry and sad that she's not here to be part of our lives or to really get to know my son, her nephew whom she would have adored. Angry that I don't have a sister or built-in best friend to go to for advice, gossip, or to vent."

After Kate lost her brother, the triggers were everywhere. "I get triggered easily when we are in the car, even if I'm not driving. I get triggered by other things too, not just by cars. I get triggered by people not being kind. I get triggered by people getting upset with each other about petty things. I get upset with the callousness of the world."

While everyone's situation and triggers are different, anger does seem to have a few favorite targets.

ANGER AT FAMILY

Siblings who were parentified at any point seemed more likely to express anger directly at their immediate family. That anger that feeds on resentment and bitterness. Anger toward the family who didn't try harder. The sister-in-law who enabled the brother's drinking. The parents who pretended everything was okay.

Rita was shocked at the intensity of anger toward her mother for not helping her brother. Anger at her other siblings for making her be the glue. But none of them know that because she doesn't want to upset them and add to their pain. So the anger grows and the anger shifts.

ANGER AT THE DECEASED

"It's hard to be angry at someone who died," Kim reflected—and yet many of us keep trying.

Like many elements of grief, cause of death does factor into how we channel our anger. In my research, siblings who experienced loss caused by suicide, addiction, and some types of violent death were most often the ones grappling with anger toward the deceased.

The anger at a sibling who died by suicide—leaving you alone in the world.

The anger at a sibling who died of an overdose—screaming, "How could they be so stupid?!" into the void.

The anger at a sibling who drove in the rain or snow or late at night.

The anger at a sibling who could have gotten out of his deployment to Afghanistan but chose to go anyway.

It isn't just the cause of death that can feed this anger; it has much to do with the nature of the relationship itself. Studies have shown that when the sibling relationship is one of both strong attachment and strong anger, riddled with interpersonal conflict, grief takes on many of those same conflicting emotions. Often this conflict manifests in anger toward the deceased and difficulty letting them go. Molly, left to care for her aging father, admitted, "I'm mad! I'm mad that everyone in my family is an addict. I have these moments of anger; I get mad at Jason and I think, 'Why the fuck are you not here helping me when I need you? I need a sibling.'" In many cases, the result of this type of grief and anger makes for "a particularly difficult grief response, characterized by an initial absence of expressed grief, followed by severe grief symptoms, guilt, self-reproach, and persistent negative feelings about past experiences."[4]

Until the anger begins to clear, it's hard to find the love required to truly grieve and assimilate to the loss. Anger masks the grief, buries it, tries to suffocate it. But grief always wins in the end.

ANGER AT SOCIETY

I recently went away for the weekend with a dear friend who also lost her big brother, hers to an accidental overdose. I call these trips my "Dead Brothers Weekends," but no one seems to find that charming (yet!). We were talking about how differently we were treated by others in the aftermath of our brothers' deaths. People's responses to overdose being wildly different from how they'd view a fallen soldier.

"But do you ever get mad at just . . . society?" she asked. "Our culture? The fact that our society is, ultimately, what killed both of our brothers?"

I do. I really, really do.

Society's greed is what fuels the opioid crisis. It's what starts wars. It's what dictates that one death is dignified and the other a blight.

Our culture did this to us.

But what do you do with anger toward a concept like society? It's much easier to be mad at a face and a name. Anger toward society is what fuels Holden Caulfield, surrounded by phonies.

But Holden wasn't okay either. Anger at the phonies didn't help him. It didn't bring him peace. It didn't suffocate the grief. Grief won again.

ANGER AT THE KILLER

Sometimes there is an actual known, responsible party for our loss.

The person driving the car.

The person pulling the trigger.

The person supplying the drugs.

The person who ended another's life.

Until I conducted these interviews, I thought seeing my brother's killer brought to justice would have helped in some way. Put a fine point on my wild rage. I spoke with some siblings who saw the killer put behind bars; for some it did help. It added closure, a record, an action. Susan told me she'd been "living in a fog" for the seven years since her sister's murder. She struggled to hold a job, to sleep, to exist. When she found out the suspect would be going to trial, she told me she could breathe again. When they got a guilty verdict, she threw a party to celebrate.

Claudia barely remembers her brother's killer's trial at all and has no interest in reminders. She knows they're easily accessible. Her oldest brother still tracks the perpetrator's prison transfers and sentence status.

So I guess what I'm saying is—one person's closure is another's boogeyman.

The grief wins again.

MARIE KONDO THAT ANGER

When I would let the anger overtake me, I would often listen to "Strangers" by the Kinks on a loop. I listened to it enough that I didn't need to hear the song out loud, I could play it on demand in my mind. The song, like so many others, could express the emotions I was struggling to name and describe for myself. In it, brothers Ray and Dave Davies sing, "For many men there is so much grief. And my mind is proud but it aches with rage."

My mind is proud but it aches with rage.

It was the first time I heard anyone (including myself) so accurately describe the dichotomy of anger and love that was eating me alive. That I could be so angry at my brother and at our society, and so very proud of the life he lived and the person he was.

At the time of writing, I'm thirteen years out from my brother's death. And yet, while writing this chapter I got so angry at the injustice of it all that I gave in to a good, loud, ugly cry and primal scream. It was the scream that woke my dog from her nap, and it was her barking that snapped me out of it. As I calmed back down, breathing slowly, I realized it was no longer anger—not really. It was sadness. Sadness of a little sister who just missed her big brother. Sadness of a heartbroken sibling who only wanted a hug.

So I picked up my phone.

"Hi. I love you," I texted Sam.

"Love you!" he responded almost immediately.

And I smiled and picked up my pen. Because anger can try to suffocate my grief, but grief is a component of love, and I can finally choose to feel the love.

nine

Getting Lost in the Lost

If I ever lost my eyes / if my colors all run dry / yes if I ever
lose my eyes / oh well / I won't have to cry no more.

—Yusuf / Cat Stevens

I didn't know it was possible to be so full of emotion and feel so empty
at the same time. For my eyes to burn because my tear ducts had dried
up. I didn't know I could see his face on random passersby and struggle to
take a full breath. I didn't know about the physical pain, the sore throat,
the pounding headaches, the exhaustion. In the first few years after Ben's
death, I cried myself to sleep more often than not. I upped my Lexapro
and moved through the world mechanically, choosing to do the things
that I believed were expected of me without any consideration for what I
actually wanted.

At the time I didn't see this as a depression, though of course it was.
In my mind depression was that deep-seated sadness that was almost

inexplicable. I remember as a child there were times when I would just cry, and my dad would ask what was wrong, but all I could respond was "I don't know." That was what I considered depression—feeling the weight of the world, and the only thing I could do was curl up and cry, but I didn't know why, which made everything worse. Depression, to me, was looking at my life and thinking I have nothing to be this sad about, and yet I was sad anyway. This thing that I felt after Ben died, the weight and the tears, there was a reason. How could I not feel this sadness? How can I not feel my world crumble? My person, my biggest brother, my idol, my guide, was gone. So according to my (incorrect and harmful) understanding of mental health, this wasn't depression. This was just the world I now inhabited. This was what it would be from now on, for the rest of my life. With depression, I thought, there's treatment and something I can do—there are medications that I can take, there's therapy. But no medication or therapist was going to bring back my brother. This was my existence, and this would be my existence until I die. I was convinced the only thing that would make this better would be bringing my brother back and, as much as I like to believe in magic, I did not believe that my brother was coming back from the dead.

Now don't get me wrong, I took antidepressants and I still do, but I also believed that this was not technically "depression"—it was just being sad that your brother died. Of course, the truth is that I was in the throes of a deep and soul-crushing depression. I struggled to get out of bed, struggled to continue to go to school, cried on the subway, and rarely answered the phone.

Shortly after Ben died, my best friend and her older sister came over to help me "reorganize" (read: clean) my apartment. I'm not really sure how this plan came about except I think that I was living in filth, and they wanted to help. So they came over and we each had a job; mine was to put away the clothes that were piled on the floor in my room. As music blasted Emily reorganized my kitchen shelves, Lissa reassembled the living room, and I curled up in the fetal position on my bed and sobbed. The music was loud enough that they were oblivious for a time, reassembling my life as I cried alone. I'm not sure how long it took them to find me (it may have been two minutes or twenty), but they did find me, and they climbed into bed to envelop me. Then they did the best thing you can do in that situation: they just lay there. They asked nothing of me, but they rubbed my back and let me cry, and when I was done I took a deep breath and Emily showed me my new, beautiful, reorganized kitchen cabinets.

Severe levels of depression are all too common among grieving siblings. Studies have shown that when compared to those grieving the loss of a friend, siblings are significantly more likely to suffer from depression, and that depression is more severe.

And then it gets worse. Not only were those siblings more likely to suffer from depression, but they also had a significantly lower sense of meaningfulness in the world, benevolence in the world, and lower self-worth. Among those grieving the loss of a friend, these levels were equal to non-bereaved. But not siblings. The world had failed them, and they no longer trusted its benevolence, no longer saw the meaning of it all—the meaning of themselves.[1] As one sibling described it, the loss of his brother "really blew the lid off the vacuum chamber of meaning in my life."

I experienced this swirling despair—feeling as if I'd lost my brother and all meaning at once—but I didn't know it had a name.

Its name is anguish.

Grieving siblings experience anguish. Brené Brown defines anguish as "an almost unbearable and traumatic swirl of shock, incredulity, grief, and powerlessness."[2] This combination of emotion hits us physically and emotionally; it's what causes you to literally drop to your knees when you learn of the death. That is the feeling we're going to focus on now. Buckle up. We're going to the lowest of low, the most hopeless emotion. Anguish.

SHOCK

Shock appears in the aftermath of a loss, before grief settles in. Shock leaves you reeling; your entire world has shifted off its axis leaving you literally and figuratively off balance. Siblings told me that in those moments of acute grief, they didn't know if they—or the world—would ever feel "right" again, or if it was forever off-kilter. "How am I supposed to be?" Caity recalled asking herself. "What is the path forward?"

The shock at learning of, and adjusting to, the death of a loved one triggers a hormonal and chemical stress response. In other words, this shock triggers our fight, flight, or freeze response. For some, life simply stops. Frozen. The shock locking them in place, unable to step beyond it. Others collapse in tears. Some may scream a primal scream from deep inside. I am a freezer. Big time. Because of my frozen state (I believe), there are a lot of things about those first few weeks that I simply do not remember. It was as if I was asleep with my eyes open, sleepwalking through a dream I'd never remember. Years after my brother's death, I was talking to his best friend, Kevin, about that first weekend after it happened. He'd been at the small airport with us when Ben's body was flown in, waiting on the tarmac under the full moon. I remember the moon. I don't remember Kevin being there. I don't remember the sound that escaped my mother's mouth upon seeing her son's casket being unloaded from the airplane; but Kevin does. He described it as a sound unlike anything he'd ever heard before.

This stress response ramps up your emotions and hijacks your brain's frontal lobe—the part of your brain that handles sensible things like planning and decision-making. The way I imagine it, scientifically, is that the emotions have basically all hulked out, transformed into steroid-driven cannibals, and the rational frontal lobe is like, "Nope. I'm not going anywhere near that." Remember, I am not a scientist.

So here we are, experiencing a traumatic stress response as our emotions take over and our frontal lobe takes a backseat to everything it used to control, like rational decision-making and planning for the future. And this shock isn't isolated to the moment you learned of your sibling's death. The shock follows you every day in the weeks that follow. Every time you're reminded of the loss or grappling to learn the new vocabulary. Experiencing this stress response over and over begins to rewire your brain through a process called neuroplasticity.

Then there comes a moment when your eyes start to focus again, and it appears as if everyone else's world has returned to "normal" while yours falls further and further askew. Your new neural pathways are not yet created, and your brain searches around for detours to connect synapses that were once so strong. But no one can see that. This is the moment when we, as siblings, are expected to return to normal. Our time to grieve has ended. The moment, which came up time and time again in my work, when the support that showed up that first week, first month, has left. They return to their lives and you're alone.

Truly. Painfully. Unwittingly. Alone.

You're alone with a brain that is being driven by intense emotions that really shouldn't be allowed to drive.

The feeling of isolation, the depth of which left many reeling, isn't discussed enough. Many who experienced it expressed shame or a self-image of selfishness. The drive to appear okay kicks into gear, and we bury the feelings of isolation and sorrow. In order to combat that isolation, we need to be honest—with ourselves and with others. Unless you're surrounded by mind-readers, other people will not understand the chaos going on within your brain—both literally and figuratively. You need to be okay with asking for help, company, support, anything. We all need someone, anyone, to ask how we are doing. We need to accept that talking about it isn't what makes it true. It's true whether we like it or not.

INCREDULITY

Because that frontal lobe was the part of our brain that once allowed us to imagine the future and comprehend abstract concepts, its absence makes it nearly impossible to comprehend any new reality. Even those who cared for their sibling through extended illness and experienced anticipatory grief reported shock and incredulity when death actually won out. One sister told me of sitting at her big sister's bedside as she battled cancer. The night she passed, she remembered, "I was sitting next to her, holding her hand watching her every breath. I remember she breathed in, and I waited for the next exhale and inhale pattern, but it never came. I always pictured these moments to be like the movies and TV shows where monitors start alarming, and doctors come rushing. But that didn't happen. I frantically woke up my parents and called for someone to come. How could she be gone? I wasn't ready to let go yet." As someone who experienced a sudden death, I admit I was surprised at her confusion. I had mistakenly assumed that the "how could they be gone?" feeling (i.e., incredulity) was isolated to sudden death. It's not. Remember, our rational brain has left the building at this point—we're running purely on emotional fuel.

For those who were unable to view their sibling's body, for whatever reason, the incredulity was even more pervasive. Seeing is believing after all, and if you don't see it, it's much easier to believe it isn't real.

The Army strongly advised us not to open the casket or view the remains. Jews don't embalm or do open-casket, so I'd never expect to see a family member displayed after death, but not being able to identify the remains fueled my incredulity. How do I know what's in that coffin? Am I supposed to just . . . believe you? YOU? The institution responsible for this nightmare? I'm supposed to trust you now? Not likely. I'll believe it when I see it. We all know that, logically, a refusal to accept the truth does not change the fact that it is true; but when emotions are running the brain-show, that logic is very literally not accessible.

POWERLESSNESS

Anguish doesn't only live in the brain; it has physical traits and implications resulting in a feeling of powerlessness over our own bodies.

Anguish is what caused my knees to buckle when Sam told me what happened.

Anguish is what made Jessica double over on the side of the highway as her mother told her of her sister's overdose and her two young children watched from the backseat.

Anguish is what caused Ryan's muscle tension and night sweats.

Anguish is why Andrew began suffering from panic attacks.

Anguish, as Brown describes, "comes for our bones."[3]

But bones aren't all it's after because anguish is a greedy little bastard. Anguish also comes for our mind—leaving us utterly powerless. This is where, in my observations, the sense of meaninglessness takes over. Our minds resign.

Among many women I spoke with, the feeling of powerlessness caused them to shut down. As if their will crumpled to the floor along with their bodies at the moment their knees gave out. Caity drew the comparison to the adults in the *Peanuts* cartoons, knowing people are talking, but it comes out like unintelligible sounds, not actual words. "I wouldn't be looking at whoever was talking, but I didn't hear a fucking thing that they said to me. I didn't even know if I was nodding my head and pretending I understood what they were saying. I didn't even care." She described it as being both numb and in excruciating pain.

While the exact cause is unknown, studies have shown that depression can manifest differently in men than women. In addition to the feelings of sadness, hopelessness, and melancholy that may be experienced during depression, men are more likely to exhibit behavioral symptoms that aren't always recognized as depression. These include escapist behavior, substance abuse, increased risky behavior, physical symptoms (headaches, etc.), and anger. After Andrew's brother died, he told me, "I literally couldn't function. I was already drinking plenty before that, but it accelerated afterward. And that meaninglessness . . . truly not giving a fuck if I woke up the next morning because . . ." He feigned incredulity and looked around as he called out, "Am I stuck on earth with all these assholes?" He shook his head. "Fuck! Send me wherever Paul is, you know, I don't care if it's hell. At least I'll be there with him."

Reading back over my interview with Andrew, I couldn't help but think of my new friend, Holden Caulfield, stuck in a world full of phonies who couldn't hold a candle to his brother. Like Holden, many of the men I spoke to (more than nonmales) reported an increase in dangerous and/or addictive behavior during their phase of acute grief. For them, the powerlessness allowed something else to take over.

Andrew recounted developing his own addiction after his brother's death. It was something he'd been trying to understand himself while going through recovery. "I think that some part of my subconscious, the

deep, dark, really fucking dark, recesses of my brain," he laughed sardoni-
cally, "I think I wanted to go through what my brother had. I did become
an alcoholic for a while; I went through that fucking misery like some
sort of sick, twisted experiment. What a weird, hellish empathy, right?
Like, what the fuck was I doing? It's something only Paul and I would do
for each other. But it's funny I guess; it's really, really fucking twisted. I
get that, I know."

Long after our conversation, Andrew's words "a weird, hellish empathy" continued to haunt me. It's not something that Andrew, or any of us,
had any power over. As our brains began to rewire, neurons forging new
pathways and language, it tried to make sense of the senseless in ways we
didn't understand—but that felt like the only option.

LOSS OF IDENTITY

Grief is the fuel that keeps this anguish train running. The complex network of emotions for us to get lost in. There's the loss of the individual,
and there are all the network offshoots, reroutes, dead ends.

The loss of our family.

Our future.

Our memories.

Our meaning.

Our safety.

Our identity.

As we've established, much of our identities are formed by and around
our siblings. When we lose those building blocks, those foundational
stones laid by our siblings, we are forced to rebuild our identities.[4] Forced
to become a new person we don't want to be.

I don't want my identity to be the girl with a dead brother. I also don't
want my identity to be the girl with one brother. I want to be the girl with
two brothers and no fear that someone will ask a follow-up question. I
just want to be the girl with two brothers and no qualifiers.

Two brothers. Full stop.

Ryan's brother was the only one who understood her. She grieves her link to her culture. "In our twenties, we were both trying to figure out our identities, especially what it means to be Asian American in the US and how we hold on to our family traditions and our roots while also trying to fit in in the US," she explained. "It was a struggle for both of us, but also, it was a way we could bond and have those really meaningful conversations. In college he studied Mandarin, and he studied abroad in China and majored in Asian studies, so I felt like he was always my link and my passageway to feeling more connected. I didn't study Mandarin into adulthood, and I just didn't feel that connection like he did. Now that he's gone, I feel like a part of that is lost because he was so much of that tie for me."

Sharae saw her brother as the Black male role model in her children's lives, especially for her son: "I don't know how I'm going to replace that." She grieves lost opportunities for her brother to guide her son's identity development the same way he had for her.

THE ANGUISH CYCLE

Grief can continue to trigger anguish for the rest of our lives, whether through small moments of remembering or milestones that get you every. Damn. Time.

For me, that trigger is anticipatory grief.

In that first year, the grief around each milestone, birthday, holiday, and moment could set off a new, all-encompassing wave of anguish. Siblings I spoke to who were less than one year out from their losses were living deep in these moments. Barely surviving as they go through the motions and travel from one first to the next.

I survived the first Thanksgiving without him. His birthday, my birthday, graduation, and the Fourth of July. And in the years that followed, some got easier—I can eat his favorite pumpkin pie again—and others still bring me to my knees. The weird thing is, while part of me knows exactly when these moments will come, they can still surprise me. Here's a common scene in my house:

I find myself slipping into depression and will remark to my husband that I don't know why this dark cloud has settled—unable to identify the root cause.

Him: Well, today is [insert date in mid-late September].

Me: Oh. Yeah. I think I miss Ben.

Cue tears. And scene.

I struggle the most with the anniversary of his death and his birthday. Both of these events fall within the month of October, the second and twenty-second, respectively, and the anticipatory grief means that I can now reliably expect the anguish to take a crowbar to my kneecaps some-time in mid-September.

Here's how it works:

Step 1:	On or around September 15, start getting calendar invites for meetings happening on October 2.
Step 2:	Sob uncontrollably. Debate whether I should take the day off. Decide I can control it this year. I hold the power.
Step 3:	Invitations for October 1, 2, and 3 continue to roll in, each prompting a new wave of anguish.
Step 4:	Fixate on the day—what I'll do, whom I'll tell.
Step 5:	Three to five days prior to the anniversary, have a major sobbing meltdown with a 70 percent chance of a panic attack (down from 100 percent during years one to five).
Step 6:	My husband gears up to become the primary parent, giving me all the space and time I need to be alone, or the comfort of being together. Cry myself to sleep the night before.
Step 7:	Survive the day. That's it. That's the goal.
Step 8:	Wake up October 3 empty but solid, a shell of a human for sure, but able to breathe again.
Step 9:	Repeat October 4–22 ahead of his birthday.
Step 10:	Wake up October 23 and think, "I did it."

The thing I've learned is that it's best not to deny it. I'm here to remind you that you don't have to be strong every moment of every day. It's okay to wallow in your sadness. Take a deep breath and stop pretending you're okay. Stop pretending to believe that everyone else's grief is more important than your own. Stop pretending you should be "over it" by now.

Those are limiting beliefs that will only come back to bite you in the ass. Instead, think of things you can do when the anguish returns. Learn the vocabulary to express it so that if you choose to share the load, you can allow others a glimpse into your struggle.

ten

Radical Acceptance, or the Lessons of Mr. Magorium

Take it easy, but take it.

—Woody Guthrie

I'm about to say something that may be controversial.

Mr. Magorium's Wonder Emporium is the most underrated movie of all time.

You're probably asking yourself, "What is *Mr. Magorium's Wonder Emporium*?" I rest my case.

Mr. Magorium's Wonder Emporium is a 2007 film (it's not a movie; it's a film) starring Dustin Hoffman, Natalie Portman, and Jason Bateman. Now you're really wondering why you've never heard of it—it's because life isn't fair and no one appreciates true art. Mr. Magorium (played by Hoffman) is an eccentric 246-year-old owner of a magical toy store who has decided it is his time to leave this world. You see, when Magorium found the perfect pair of shoes, he purchased enough pairs to last him the rest of his life; now he is on his last pair. He tries explaining this to Molly Mahoney (Portman), his trusted employee, and she is having none of it. In a particularly poignant moment, Molly asks Mr. Magorium if he is dying, to which he responds, "Light bulbs die, my sweet. I will depart."

I repeated that line in my head dozens of times after I first heard it; it seemed like a very poetic way to think about death. At the time, death was a more distant concept for me. As of 2007, I had lost two grand-parents who were very dear to me, but they had both been in their mid-nineties and ailing. The remainder of my family—nuclear and extended—was alive and well. I had no idea that over the next two years I would lose my remaining two grandparents, one uncle, and my oldest brother.

In the wake of Ben's death, I heard Mr. Magorium's voice in my head often, but it never quite fit. To "depart" sounds calm, elegant, even cel-ebratory. Mary Poppins departed on her floating umbrella. I watched Hoffman over and over again, reciting the lines I once found so poetic and beautiful, and all I could feel was resentment. Ben's "departure" was sudden, violent, and traumatic—a bomb, both literally and figuratively. There was nothing light about the way Ben left this world, and the result-ing weight that I carry is one that won't go away. The weight is often invisible to others, but not to me—or to you. We move forward and try to rebuild our lives, but just because we carry the weight doesn't mean it isn't heavy.

Perhaps Mr. Magorium was allowed to depart because he was 246 years old; my brother was thirty-two. I believe my ninety-six-year-old grandfather departed this world, but that doesn't feel right for a thirty-two-year-old, and many whom I've spoken to feel the same.

When you lose a sibling you lose a peer, and so when your life contin-ues and theirs does not, it is a constant reminder that theirs was cut short. You were supposed to live life together; you were supposed to live for the same amount of time. The loss of a sibling, no matter how "peaceful" (lol) their departure, is known to be especially distressing, and it is common for the surviving sibling to feel as if a piece of them has died.

Not surprisingly, the physical implications of the death can be even more pronounced in twins. Harriet told me that she and her brother Seb:

> embodied the whole twin stereotype. Seb was thirty minutes older than me and took this as a sign that he was my protector. We did everything together. When he was gone, I felt like someone had chopped off my legs. I kept texting and emailing him. I kept ringing him. There was no answer but I felt there should be. And I swear I felt it happen. I know it sounds weird, but I felt my whole body drop when he died. I wasn't there and I didn't get to say goodbye.

I felt like someone had chopped off my legs.
This type of loss holds an element of violence, regardless of the cir-cumstances surrounding the death itself. I don't mean violence in its literal sense, though, yes, my brother's death was extremely violent, but sibling loss is violent in that it is unpredictable and it is unnatural. Even those who lose a sibling after a long illness will feel a sense of violence in that this person was torn from their life too soon. For that reason, some siblings who have also lost a parent observed that the loss of a sibling was harder to process and survive. One sibling described the difference as los-ing someone you love versus losing a part of yourself.

Many mourners who have lost siblings to addiction have told me that although they knew this was always a possibility, and in fact a probability, somehow the death still shocked them. They felt it like a sucker punch delivered by a metal fist covered in nails. It is violence, and it's hard to feel any peace with that kind of a loss.

When death involves violence—at the hands of the deceased or another—there is an increased chance that the bereaved will experience traumatic grief. As a reminder, traumatic grief is the combined experience of grief and PTSD. Siblings are at an increased risk of traumatic grief based on cause of death, suddenness of death, if they witnessed the death, whether they blame themselves, and their level of attachment to the deceased. Violence, specifically, is correlated to experiencing traumatic grief. The more violent the death, the higher the likelihood of experiencing traumatic grief.[1] For me, Breanne, and many others, this traumatic grief often manifested in the form of nightmares. On top of the deep trauma and issues that arise from PTSD nightmares, one common sentiment was sadness. Sadness that their sibling only appeared in nightmares. Sadness that they couldn't conjure good dreams. Sadness that the trauma was all they could feel.

I AM MORTAL

Because siblings are supposed to be our longest relationship and partner in old age, their death serves as a loud wake-up call for our own mortality. Interestingly, this reckoning happened with almost every sibling I spoke to regardless of age or cause of death. Stephanie was fifteen when her brother died of AIDS in 1991. She told me that for months after Andy's death she was haunted by a constant thought that "I'm definitely going to die too. If he could die, then I'm going to die." She explained, "Every time our car took a different turn, or somebody hit the breaks, I just kept feeling like, 'Here it is. I'm ready. I'm ready to die.' I was really making peace with death, and I saw it everywhere, and I definitely felt like I was not going to live the summer out. I just felt like I was going to die too."

This fear isn't necessarily that you die the same way, but that death is imminent. That way, you really would have lived your full lifetimes together.

Studies on sibling loss with adult siblings showed that the surviving siblings experienced a shift in their sense of self, accompanied by feelings of emptiness and hopelessness, along with (you guessed it) a fear of dying.[2] This fear is felt at all ages, even by our dear Holden, who wrote of walking up Fifth Avenue, convinced each time he stepped off a curb that he wouldn't make it to the other side. Death has robbed them of any sense of safety, and as a result, surviving siblings may assume their own early death is an unfortunate foregone conclusion—a matter of when, not if. As a result, this new realization manifested itself in the form of phobias and/or fixations with death. Siblings reported developing phobias around driving, being alone, loud noises, and sudden death, just to name a few.

After Claudia's brother was killed by an intruder in his apartment, her sense of security was taken. Rationally, she told herself that the same crime would not befall two kids in the same family, but logic has no place here. She was afraid to live alone, overthinking every sound at night, a constant fear in the pit of her stomach. Now, over twenty years later, and with a family of her own, Claudia admitted that she felt safest during the Covid-19 lockdowns because her family was home; she knew where they were and no one was alone.

Not being able to imagine how your life can continue after the loss of a sibling makes sense because in many cases, you cannot remember ever living without them. You don't know what living without them would even look like. You fear a life without them because it is not a life you've ever known. There is no evidence that you even can live without them, regardless of whether you want to or not. For this reason, most younger siblings expressed exceptionally high distress when they became older than their sibling. Remember how I tried to skip my thirty-third birthday? I wasn't the only one.

Then there are the fears that you *will* die the same way as your sibling, and this fear often surrounds experiences of addiction, suicide, and genetic illness. One sibling explained, "Although I wasn't best friends with my brother, we were still genetically linked, so thinking that something could happen to him means it could also happen to me. I've never experienced suicidal ideation, but the reality that he dealt with it for so long and succumbed to it scares me deeply and often makes me wonder if there's something inside me that will come out that would ever lead me to think those things."

Something inside me that will come out.

The fear isn't rooted in the relationship itself—it doesn't matter if you were close with your sibling or not—what matters is the biological bond and reality of genetics.

FEAR OF LOSING OTHERS

For those whose siblings died in accidents or unexplainable circumstances, there is often a fear of losing additional loved ones. When you live in the ripple of a random occurrence—whether it be a carjacking or a brain aneurysm—the world becomes a completely senseless place. Ryan's brother was an excellent swimmer. It makes no logical sense that he would drown while swimming laps. If it could happen to him, it could happen to anyone.

The fear of additional loss is not isolated to the acute phase of grief. Oh no, my friends, this one can last a lifetime. Siblings affected by addiction and mental health issues live in fear of their own children inheriting those same struggles. Cara didn't have children of her own when her brother died, and yet one of the issues she has been working through in therapy is a fear of losing a child of her own. "How will I get through that? I had a lot of fear around how I would manage if my child died, and I don't know why it's kind of come out that way. Maybe it's from seeing my parents so upset. I am pregnant right now, and when my child is born, I don't have control over if they die or not. They could die in a million different ways. Same with me, and I just have to be fine with it."

I struggled with the same fear after my son Archie was born. You might be thinking, "But, Annie, your brother was killed by a suicide bomber in an active war zone. Your toddler is not in a war zone."

And to that I would respond, "HAVE YOU LEARNED NOTHING?"

Grief—and the fears, traumas, and phobias it gives life to—is not rational! One cannot simply apply logic to a grief response. My mother lost her firstborn child, and I was destined to do the same, logic be damned! The conviction and prevalence of this fear of losing one's own child was so common that many siblings told me it was their deciding factor when determining how many children to have themselves. If they had a third child, then should something happen to one of them, no one was left alone. This is something I've thought about many, many (many) times myself. A puzzle for which there's no correct solution, no finite number of pieces. Do you plan for the worst, or do you hope for the best?

The weight of those feelings, of feeling like you need to have a third child so none are left alone should one die, is the perfect encapsulation of the weight surviving siblings carry around. The weight that impacts each and every decision we make.

ACCEPTANCE

I struggled a lot with the word "acceptance" and the notion that in order to move forward after a loss we must come to a place of "acceptance." Is it a matter of semantics? Perhaps, but words matter. For me, the word "acceptance" feels consensual. You accept a job, colleges accept students, clubs accept members; to experience "acceptance" is often a good thing. You've made it! You're in! I did not *consent* to this. I have been accepted into a club that, no offense (because I know you're in it too), is a terrible club. I realize that acceptance has other definitions, and that one of those is tolerating a difficult situation, but that's not the definition I think of when I hear that word. And so, yes, it is a matter of semantics, but I maintain—words matter.

My brother knew he could die in Afghanistan. He knew it was much more dangerous than he ever let on, and he knew that what he was doing was life-threatening. He entered that situation consensually, and perhaps he had reached a level of acceptance of the inevitability of his death; but not me. I didn't make that choice, and if faced with it again I would still fight to keep him home. Maybe that's why I struggled to experience resilient grief. Maybe if his consent had been something we shared, I could feel at peace with it, but I didn't.

Rather than "acceptance," what I felt most about my brother's death was resignation. I got to a place where I no longer denied its truth, or deluded myself with the idea that the army was wrong and he'll just come knocking on our door one day. I was resigned to the reality that he is gone from this physical world, and I am committed to living in this world without him present. But acceptance was never the word I'd use to describe it, and the more other people told me that the key to moving on was "acceptance," the more I resisted it. I did not want to accept it; I did not want to be okay with his death; I did not want to lump it in with my acceptance to college or a deposit acceptance at my local bank. For me, saying I needed to reach "acceptance" was just as bad as saying, "Everything happens for a reason"—it would cause a knee-jerk reaction and a small voice inside me would yell, "Acceptance?! I'LL SHOW YOU ACCEPTANCE!" Then I swiftly self-sabotage and prove just how non-accepting I can be about my big brother's murder.

I delivered this very argument against the word "acceptance" to Dr. Katharine Bernstein, a licensed clinical psychologist and member of our club. I expected her to laud my perspective and join me in the rally against the word "acceptance." Instead, she smiled and calmly said, "Acceptance does not equal approval—it's the acknowledgment of fact. Think of it more as 'reality acceptance' instead of a blanket acceptance; it's acknowledging that this is your reality."

Oh. Huh. Well, shit.

"Reality acceptance," I said slowly, as much to myself as to her. "I like that. I can do that."

That's when Dr. Bernstein explained the concept of radical acceptance, a cornerstone of dialectical behavior therapy (DBT) that she uses in her own practice. Radical acceptance and DBT were developed in the late 1980s by Dr. Marsha Linehan and teach distress tolerance and reality acceptance. She has stated, "Radical acceptance rests on letting go of the illusion of control and a willingness to notice and accept things as they are right now, without judging." Linehan believes that suffering is the result of pain *plus* nonacceptance, and this suffering can be avoided through acceptance. The pain exists in both scenarios; it's what you do with it that makes all the difference.[3]

The "radical" in radical acceptance means you are all in—there's no selective acceptance. It means not only accepting the reality that your sibling has died, but also accepting the deep anguish you feel and all the ripple effects of grief. Accepting those things without judgment is essential; accept that you feel sad without berating yourself; accept that you're angry without a disclaimer; accept whatever emotion it is you are feeling and allow yourself to really feel it without self-judgment. It's about feeling the emotion, not resisting it or trying to bury it away, without trying to *fix* anything. This will not be easy, none of this is easy—it is a practice. We need to practice radical acceptance every day in all aspects of our lives, but especially in this one.

Dr. Tara Brach is a clinical psychologist and meditation teacher as well as the author of the book *Radical Acceptance: Embracing Your Life with the Heart of a Buddha*. Brach teaches that one way to approach radical acceptance is by practicing RAIN.[4]

R—Recognize what is happening.

A—Allow the experience to be there, just as it is.

I—Investigate with interest and care.

N—Nurture with self-compassion.

A is the hardest one for me. Okay, fine, A through N are all pretty far out of my comfort zone. Giving space to hard emotions and not running from them—letting them exist "just as it is" without trying to fix or bury them—will be a lifelong practice for me. And self-compassion . . . I am not good at self-compassion. I don't even like sitting in silence for fear of what my brain might say to me. This is an ongoing practice for me too, but with time and patience, that little voice is already more generous and accepting of me. I think we might be becoming friends. What you call it doesn't matter. Radical acceptance, reality acceptance, inner beast—it doesn't matter. What matters is that once you reach that place of radical acceptance [or insert your magic word here], the grief shifts and begins to take on new forms, and you begin to see opportunities for continued connection and presence in this new reality. You still feel pain, but that's okay. You don't judge yourself for it, and you learn to integrate it into your reality. That's when we open up to the possibilities of joy.

Part III

Within

eleven

Joy Grief

Do you realize / that happiness makes you cry? / Do you realize / that everyone you know someday will die?

—The Flaming Lips

It's time to take a deep breath, open the curtains, and venture into the great unknown. That unknown, of course, being life without our sibling's physical presence. I stress physical because the key to all of this, to our continued bonds, is in developing the ability to feel their presence in other ways. To reestablish the relationship and learn to live with them inside our hearts and minds in whatever way is healthy and beneficial for us. But before we focus on *us* we need to focus on *you*. You're the one walking a new path, and you are central to this story. It's easy to forget that you're the main character in your own life, isn't it? It's not about your siblings, parents, or anyone else. Not right now.

The first time I felt true joy in the months after Ben's death, it was followed by a wave of depression that I had never anticipated. I hadn't felt joy, true happiness, in so long that I didn't think those kinds of highs were even possible. Then when it happened, it was as if I had finally made it to the top of the tower of terror, only to plunge back down again.

There is an aftershock to joy when you can't share it with your person. There is a unique feeling of guilt, that you shouldn't be allowed to feel happy without them, accompanied by that oh-so-friendly reminder that you will never hear the voice of the person whose voice mirrors your own. How dare I feel joy when my brother is (still) dead? Selfish little sister, brat, heartless—take your pick. I didn't believe I was worthy or deserving of joy and, as we covered in previous chapters, god help anyone who dares tell you that your sibling "would have wanted you to be happy." Oh no. No, no, no. They would have wanted to share your happiness with you in person, not from their seat in the afterlife where they're definitely yelling at you to see all of the signs they've been waving in your face already (but we'll get to that).

It's not just your own joy that can topple into sadness, but the recognition of all the things your sibling will never experience. Getting married wasn't just hard because Ben wouldn't be there to stand under the chuppah and give a toast berating my husband, but because he never got to have a wedding himself. When my oldest son was born, I wept not only because my son would never meet his uncle, but because Ben never got to have kids of his own.

Beth's older brother was killed in a car crash when they were teenagers, and she explained that "my grief has taken different shapes over the past thirty-six years, and sometimes parts of it are almost as raw as when it happened. What would have been his high school graduation, seeing my friends' older siblings graduate college, get married, becoming aunts and uncles. That absence at my own wedding; not meeting his nieces and nephews . . . I've lived so much more of my life without my brother than with him—but that absence has never diminished."

THE TERROR OF JOY

Looking back, I think that even more than the guilt and self-loathing, I resisted joy because it terrified me. It was a reminder of how fleeting everything is. The thing that brought such joy one day could be ripped away the next. If I didn't feel joy, I couldn't feel pain. What a sad way to exist in this world, constantly muting the most beautiful moments out of fear. I suppose I shouldn't have been surprised, then, when I learned that joy is the most vulnerable emotion—more than shame or fear.[1] Joy is felt so deeply and physically that it brings some people to tears. To feel anything that deeply is risky, but especially joy. If you don't experience pure joy, then you can't have it ripped from you; if the joy is temporary, then avoiding it means avoiding the fallout. You can't miss something you never had. But here's the truth: a life without the vulnerability of joy may seem easier, but it's empty. It's vulnerability that helps us build resilience and strength—and those are the things we need most.

This is the moment when you groan and say, "She's going to make me be vulnerable and feel joy, isn't she?"

Ding ding ding ding ding!

Let's back up. What is joy exactly, and why can something so pure and bright cause such turmoil? Joy is that deep happiness you feel at your core, deep enough to bring someone to tears or change a life. While happiness can be felt as a mood or state of being, joy is acute. It is often triggered suddenly, and it involves connection—to ourselves and to others. It's watching your best friend marry their person, holding your child for the first time, or (in my case) making my kids laugh so hard they snarf. It's no wonder such a strong emotion rooted in connection could be so triggering.

If your sibling is the person you'd turn to, the person on the other end of the connection, then of course joy itself becomes a trigger when that connection is severed! In this new world, joy reminds us of what is no longer possible. We can't pick up the phone and call or text them; our arms feel empty with nothing to hold; *we* may feel empty.

Then there's the guilt—AGAIN.

[shakes fist]

Guilt that you're experiencing joy and they aren't—can't—experiencing it with you.

Guilt that you're feeling any positive emotion at all rather than living in the sadness of loss.

"How can I feel joy at a time like this?" may be running through your head. And to that I say, "A time like *what*?!" This is it; this is the only time we have. There is no other timeline, no options. You know what I think? I think "a time like this" is an excuse I used for a long time to avoid being vulnerable; pretending to be all noble; refusing to feel joy when my brother was gone and more were dying every day wasn't noble. I was just trying to avoid the extreme ends of the emotional spectrum because I didn't want to feel that level of pain ever again, and if giving up joy could help avoid that—then that's what I'd do. I wish I could go back in time, flag down younger Annie, and scream in her face, "Don't shut yourself off to joy! Being happy doesn't mean you're happy about Ben's death, it just means you're allowing yourself to live!" Then I'd cover her in glitter.

I know now, after speaking with so many siblings, that I'm not the only one who tried to resist joy. In my research, this resistance was most common in the first five years after a sibling's death, or as a manifestation of longer-lasting, complicated grief. One sibling, who was only one year out from her sister's death, explained, "I still have this limiting belief that if I let the grief pass through me, I have to let Laurie go too. So I'm fiercely holding on to my grief."

Fiercely holding on to my grief.

When your arms are so full of grief, when each finger is clinging to it, nails dug in, you can't hold any joy. You can't hold anything else at all. It reminds me of the children's book *Hershel and the Hanukkah Goblins*, in which (spoiler alert) the king of the goblins gets his hand stuck in a pickle jar when he refuses to let go of the pickles in his fist. The goblin's hand would continue to be trapped in that jar until he made the decision to let go of the pickles. You see where I'm going with this. Don't cling to your grief so tightly that you can't experience the joy of eating pickles.

Some siblings, especially those who experienced resilient grief, seemed to naturally understand that living with joy was a way to honor their siblings who no longer walked this earth. Others still acknowledged this on a rational level but put in significant work to get to the point where they could actually practice and experience it. As Sarah put it, "You can't get out of depression if you can't let yourself be happy—you need to reach out for help and put in the work." The good news is that your relationship with joy isn't fixed. With time it will come back, if you allow it to.

Letting in joy can be something of a dance . . .

Joy—two steps forward

Loneliness—one step back

Joy—two steps forward

Guilt—one step back

But as we learn and grow, the dance begins to smooth out until we can learn to share our joy in new ways and allow those setbacks to become a natural part of the dance.

I got married about two and a half years after Ben died. Two steps forward.

We had a very small wedding, and no wedding party, because I couldn't fathom one without him. One step back.

Ben loved a celebratory cigar, so in his honor we had a cigar-rolling station—two steps forward.

WHEN FORGIVENESS ISN'T POSSIBLE

This ability to feel joy in relation to your sibling is not possible for everyone. For some, especially those with strained relationships or who lost their sibling to addiction or suicide, it can be a much more complex dance. Laura told me, "I often think about if my brother were alive today, to see the birth of my son and potentially have a relationship with my son . . . would that be a good thing?"

So much of what we experience in our grief is a reflection of what we felt in that relationship throughout our lives. Death doesn't wipe the slate clean; it doesn't excuse the hurt, rewrite history, or serve as a blanket apology. Often it's the opposite. Death robs us of any faint hope of reconciliation; it robs us of the future. Some people may tell you to forgive the dead, that holding onto pain and resentment won't serve you and forgiveness will bring you "peace." I'm not convinced.

Some actions and behaviors don't warrant blanket forgiveness. Don't believe me? Rabbi Elliot Kukla, a hospice rabbi who has sat by many a deathbed helping family members navigate the maze that is grieving an estranged or toxic family member, put it this way: "It's simply not true that blood is the ultimate bond; some families have become so damaged by trauma that time together is harmful for all involved."[2] Instead, Rabbi Kukla advocates for the understanding and acceptance that not all endings are happy, and death rarely puts a nice car dealership bow on any relationship.

When I was in fifth grade, a girl in my class broke my devil sticks. Stick with me here. . . . So Susan broke my devil sticks just as I was starting to get good at juggling them, and I was *furious*. After pulling us aside in the hallway, our teacher explained that Susan owed me an apology, but I did not owe her my forgiveness. My ten-year-old mind exploded. As a people-pleasing youngest child, I had never considered that forgiveness was a gift I could bestow on someone—or not—at my discretion. Drunk on my new sense of power, I told Susan I'd need to think about it. That was it! Our teacher didn't try to tell me all the reasons why it was an accident or guilt me into forgiving—he accepted that I needed time and gave it to me.

If you were estranged from, or had an otherwise difficult relationship with, your sibling, there's likely a good reason for that. Their death does not automatically warrant forgiveness, it does not symbolize that apology you've been waiting for, and it doesn't erase the past. You do not owe anyone your forgiveness. For some, this is the hardest part—pushed by a society that seems to believe we should grant blanket absolution to anyone with an apology, you might feel like a monster for not forgiving your sibling. You are not a monster. Some things don't warrant forgiveness, and you are the only one who can make that decision.

MOVING FORWARD (OR BEING THE MOST HUMAN)

It may feel like resisting joy makes things easier—without the accompanying vulnerability we may feel safe inside our protective shell, but that shell also blocks any path to resilience and strength. Remember—resilience is the name of the game here. We have no control over what happened, and we cannot change it. All we can control is how we move forward, grow, and respond to this new world.

But HOW?!

[shakes fist again; so many shaking fists]

The first step to building resilience is to take a moment to notice and appreciate what we have. Seriously—do it now. Close your eyes and think of three things you're grateful for. Be as specific as possible. Do you feel the shift? The best way to combat foreboding joy is to focus on what we *do* have, rather than bracing for the worst. Let's appreciate the goodness right here. For me that can take many forms, but when it comes to Ben, the thing I try to focus on is that I got to have my biggest brother for twenty-five full, beautiful years. I'm grateful for the time we spent as a trio, and I'm grateful for every moment I get to spend with Sam as a duo. I feel pain and sadness even writing that because I still feel I *should* have had him much longer, and we *should* still be a trio, but those twenty-five years were a gift, and I try to remember that each day.

I've recently become fascinated by people who express gratitude for grief. Yes—gratitude for grief. Stephen Colbert and Molly Shannon are both members of our esteemed Dead Siblings Club and have spoken about their losses extensively. Colbert's father and two of his brothers were killed in a plane crash when he was ten years old, and Shannon's mother, cousin, and younger sister were killed in a car crash when she was only four years old. In a 2019 interview with Anderson Cooper (also a member of the club), Colbert explains his gratitude this way:

> I want to be the most human I can be, and that involves acknowledging and ultimately being grateful for the things that I wish didn't happen because they gave me a gift.[3]

Cooper seems genuinely confused by, and curious about, this perspective. Decades out from the loss of his own brother, Cooper hasn't reached a point of gratitude. Later in the interview, Colbert notes,

> It's like living with a beloved tiger and it's that feeling, it's that grief. When I say grateful for it, I don't want to say that it's no longer a tiger. It is. And it can really hurt you. It can surprise you, it can pounce on you in moments that you don't expect—or at least that's my experience and I can't speak for everybody, but it's my tiger and I wouldn't want to get rid of the tiger. I have such a relationship with it now. I want to be clear that it's painful and it's going to live as long as I do, but that there's some symbiotic relationship between me and this particular pain that I've made peace with. So I don't regret the existence of it. That again, does not mean I wish it had ever become my tiger.

Y'all, listen—I'm not there yet. I'm trying every day and I know I've made huge strides. If you're not there yet, not even close, that's okay. One day at a time.

Joy and gratitude are two of the things we don't talk about. How would it sound to others to say we're grateful for grief? Especially us siblings—diminished in our grief from day one, fighting to be acknowledged. We may think expressing gratitude makes it seem like we're grateful for the death, but *it does not*. As Jules said of her brother's death, "It made me realize you need to embrace life and make the most of it. I made it to sixty and he never got that opportunity, so I need to embrace it and enjoy it."

CONNECTING WITH OTHERS

This is the moment when you might be thinking, "Okay, I get that joy and gratitude are good *in theory*, but it doesn't apply to me. I'm the exception to the rule." Guess again, my friend! There are many ways in which we can begin to feel joy and gratitude, none of which diminish our love for our siblings or make their deaths frivolous. The key element, I've found, is connection. Joy thrives in connection; it loves to be shared and passed back and forth; joy makes us *want* to connect and share.

Leading up to the ten-year anniversary of my brother's death, I had few connections left to his people. I had my own friends from childhood who knew him, but I had lost touch with his best friends—those four boys who practically lived at our house when I was in elementary school. I had spoken to a few of his army buddies after his death, but the conversations were brief and strained, and most had quickly fallen out of touch with our family. I realized that each of those people held a kernel of Ben within them; each knew something about him that I didn't; each carried him with them in a different way. I was feeling greedy, and I wanted them to share their kernels with me. At this point I was nearly a decade into my career as an ethnographic researcher who collects stories for a living. Could I do that same thing here? I could.

First I told Sam, pitching him my idea over dinner. "It's a great idea, but can you really do it?" he asked. "Like, can you hear all those stories? I think it would destroy me."

"I can. And if it gets to be too much, I'll stop," I assured him.

"You're a strong woman. I say do it. Maybe we can even make the interviews into a podcast."

Next I told my parents, sending them an email so that they could read and respond in their own time without being put on the spot. My dad responded later that day,

I think your idea is a wonderful one. We all know how important it is to keep Ben's memory alive and what better way than the one you have suggested. I am pretty sure we could go back even to kindergarten with Ben's teacher reports. I also have many other papers, letters, documents which would be helpful to you. We can talk in person next weekend or anytime by phone before then but your idea is a great one!

The next time I went to their house, he'd already pulled boxes of documents, letters, and records from the attic. He needed this as much as I did.

Bolstered by their faith and support, I emailed Ben's best friend and asked if he'd be my first interview. After three days of continuously refreshing my email, his response landed in my inbox:

> I'll talk about Ben anytime, anywhere. If you have questions you'd like to help guide things, send them my way. If you want me to speak extemporaneously, I can do that too. If it's some kind of mix of the two, I'm happy to go there. Whatever it may be, I'm ready to take the journey with you.
>
> Your brother's a very real presence to me. Time has never changed that. Ben's always there in the writing I do, both professionally and personally. He's there in what I say and in what I leave unsaid. In the moments between the words. The moments beyond the words. The forever moments.
>
> Talk soon,
>
> K

He wanted to take the journey *with me*. I was connected, once again, to my brother's best friend, and in that way I felt like I had been gifted a kernel of my brother. I haven't been on a first date since 2008, and I have known Kevin since I was an infant, and yet meeting up with him that morning in 2019 felt like the most stressful first date of my life. Perhaps it was because I didn't usually cry on first dates, or because I didn't usually record my first dates using a recorder and mic I'd bought on eBay, or perhaps it was because I had never had a real conversation with Kevin. Sure, I knew him, he was at my house constantly when I was a kid and he only lived a few doors down, our mothers were close friends, and he was Ben's person—but I didn't have my own relationship with him.

I set up my equipment and tested it about a dozen times before he arrived, and then there he was. My brother's person, traveling the world without my brother by his side. I almost didn't recognize him without his foil. Turns out, he didn't always recognize himself either. For the next three hours, we emptied our emotions into that little rented room on Nineteenth Street. We did all the cliché things—laughed, cried, made fun of our dads, and caught up on the past ten years. The missing ten years. Kevin loved my brother like I did, and I could see that not just in the way he spoke about their time together, but in those moments when he grappled to find the right way to express the depth of their connection. I could see it in his eyes, his hands, his nervous laugh.

He told me about their cross-country road trip, their long phone conversations in college, and the time my brother excitedly introduced him to Blues Traveler. Then he recounted the moment he heard the news that Ben had been killed, and what it was like to stand behind us on the tarmac at Tweed Airport that night. He remembered that noise my mother made.

About two hours in, once we had no real secrets left and had both cried openly, I admitted that after I left I was going to talk with a medium for the first time. I felt silly saying it out loud, but he didn't laugh at me—he wanted more. We talked about the signs we'd gotten from Ben over the years, most in the form of songs, which made sense because the man loved nothing more than a good song lyric. I promised to let him know how it went, and after many hugs and promises to continue the conversation, I got on the train back to Brooklyn.

Later that day I received an email from Kevin: "I'm in a coffee shop by Penn Station and they're playing Blues Traveler. Some days are just beautiful."

As it often happens, when I woke up that morning I did not know it was the day that would change my life. I thought I'd have an awkward conversation with Kevin, which would inevitably result in me losing my courage and abandoning the project altogether, but that didn't happen. Instead I felt joy.

That joy was invigorating and addictive; I wanted to collect all the kernels. I wanted to be connected to his people again. I wanted to form those relationships. I wanted to acknowledge and celebrate all the joy and sorrow we shared. So I kept going.

Ten months after that very first sit-down with Kevin, with five more interviews under my belt, I sat in Ben's childhood bedroom and gathered up the courage to seek out Ben's fellow service members. Some names I knew from letters they'd written us after his death and visits that first year, others I knew nothing about except what I could gather from Ben's diaries and emails. I made sure to use Ben's full name in the subject line, thinking they'd be more inclined to read the unsolicited email. Some wrote back almost immediately while others took months to reply—admitting later that they hadn't known what to say and needed the time to process the request. Some never responded and that's okay.

In that little bedroom, propped up on his bed with my laptop and (now trusty) recorder, I talked to the men who had seen a side of my brother that I never knew. Men who recounted the depths of their PTSD and survivor's guilt through clenched teeth and steady tears. Men who'd watched Ben's casket get loaded into that airplane and had to go back to work as if everything was okay. I would mute myself while they spoke as the heavy sobs wrenched my body.

One of the most surprising things I learned during these calls was that many saw my brother the same way I did. I may not have known them, but they knew Ben and they understood his power. I'm not sure who got more out of our conversations—me or them. While I gathered up all the stories and memories I could fit on that recorder, they were finally able to connect with a small piece of Ben that lived on in me, and I could tell them—without a shadow of a doubt—that none of this was their fault and that we know no one could have saved him. I could tell them that we didn't blame them. I could tell them it was going to be okay. For all the tears shed on those calls, there was an equal (or greater) amount of joy and gratitude. They reminded me that while my brother may be dead, he lived. Not only in my memories or imagination, but he really, truly lived and was witnessed.

CONNECTING WITH THE DECEASED

Finding joy in connection isn't limited to connections with the living. Yeah, you read that right (cue spooky ghost music). I believe that we can continue to feel a connection to our siblings after their death, and that connection can be incredibly soothing and joyous.

I met Sharon Cooper at a work event in 2019. She'd bravely gotten on stage in front of hundreds of women at Facebook's Women in Leadership conference and spoken about the sudden and tragic loss of her sister Sandra Bland. I began crying less than thirty seconds into her introduction. Weeks later, moved and inspired by her story, we met one-on-one over video conference, and I asked her how she'd done it. She told me about the contents of her sister's diaries, and I admitted that my brother had been an obsessive diarist who had left at least ten diaries lined up on a shelf in my parents' house before he was deployed.

"You've read them though, right?" she asked.

"No, no one has."

"No one has opened the diaries in ten years?" She seemed genuinely confused.

"Nope. I don't know if I'm supposed to. He didn't leave any instructions; I don't know if he wants me to read them."

There was silence for a moment as she stared at me before responding confidently, "If you're waiting for a sign, consider this your sign. He left them for you and you need to read them. I'm sure of it."

That night I was looking for something in my closet and spotted the two journals that I have of his. I'm not sure why I had them, but I suspect I'd found them when we were cleaning out my parents' house and grabbed them so they wouldn't get lost. I'd never opened them. I picked one up and opened it to the first page to see the date of Monday, September 4, 1984:

"Last year we went to lighthouse point at the same time my sister was born."

Message received.

Over the next six months, I collected all the diaries I could find. Our parents had moved years earlier, and the diaries were no longer lined up neatly on that shelf, but they weren't gone. Some were in Sam's attic, others in my parents', and a few from Afghanistan were packed up with the belongings that the army had returned. Each time I held a new diary in my hands, I'd devour the words as fast as I could, often making Aaron, my husband, sit there as I excitedly read excerpts aloud and we'd reminisce or draw parallels to our own children. Those diaries that I'd been so afraid of brought me such joy because they gave me new memories and a connection I didn't know was possible.

Later that year, bolstered by my newly revived connection to Ben's life and the incredible people in it, I was ready to face the ten-year anniversary of his death. "This year is going to be different," I declared to Aaron with all the confidence of a delusional toddler. "I'm not going to sit around crying; I'm going to do something."

He didn't miss a beat. "Let's plan a day Ben would have loved," he declared. "I already took the day off, and I'm all yours."

Aaron had been through it all with me. He'd met Ben when we were first dating, and in an awkward moment in the corner of our parents' kitchen, Ben had put his arm around Aaron's shoulders and from his towering height asked, "How do you intend on supporting my sister?" "Oh, I don't," Aaron replied, "she doesn't need me to." After that, Aaron became the only boyfriend Ben ever approved of. In the months after Ben's death, I'd tried to convince Aaron that he should leave me. I was useless and needy and he hadn't signed up for this. But he didn't leave. Instead, he'd stay on the phone until I cried myself to sleep, and he'd keep the line open for hours in case I woke back up. Aaron understood what I needed, often before I'd realized it myself.

On the morning of October 2, 2019, we dropped our kids off at day care and hopped on the train to South Street Seaport where we'd board the ferry to Governors Island and begin our adventure. We would rent bikes and explore, just as Ben would have done, and we'd be sure to stop at every food truck we passed. The weirder, the better. On our way home we stopped at a fancy bakery and picked up a pumpkin pie, which we ate with our kids while telling them stories about Uncle Ben.

On the ten-year anniversary of the worst moment of my life, I had a wonderful day. I had a day with Ben in which I could feel his presence more strongly and genuinely than I had in the ten years since his death. I am eternally grateful for the feeling of connection and love I felt for my brother on that day. I didn't know it was even possible to feel that kind of connection to someone who was gone, but somehow I did it. I felt joy and gratitude for my big brother, and the most remarkable thing happened: the joy and gratitude overshadowed the grief. My bucket, empty for so long, was filling back up. There was still a hole in it, but it was finally filling faster than it could drain.

If I didn't love Ben so deeply, I wouldn't feel the pain, and as much as I despise his absence and the pain it has caused, it's better than living in a world that never included him to begin with. In that way, I suppose I am starting to experience gratitude for grief.

twelve

Who Am I Now?

I'll keep on healing all the scars / that we've collected from
the start / I'd rather this than live without you.

—Eddie Vedder

The year was 1994 and ten-year-old Annie was venturing to sleep-away camp for the first time. Sam went to an all-boys camp and Ben didn't go to camp anymore, so I had to find my own way. Of course, I had no interest in finding my own way, so I'd chosen the camp where Ben's friends were counselors. I figured that if I couldn't have my brothers around, I'd have their friends. It was much less scary than going somewhere completely new where no one knew me (or my brothers). If the counselors were friends with Ben, then they'd like me because they liked him; and everyone liked him. Even at ten I knew that if I was "Ben's sister" I didn't have to prove myself—he'd already done it for all of us.

Ben had given me very clear instructions before I'd left: "You need to find Todd and AK. Tell them who you are and they'll take care of you." It was my main mission: before making friends of my own I needed to find my surrogate brothers because, as we've established, I only knew how to operate as one of three. Todd found me first, yelling, "YOU'RE A SKLAVER!" as he grabbed my face, smushing my cheeks and looking into my eyes. "It's you! You're the littlest Sklaver!"

"Yep, it's me! Annie!" I was thrilled.

"The littlest Sklaver!" He continued, "Eh, that doesn't sound right . . . We called your brothers Sklave-Dog and Sklave-Pup, so we'll call you . . . Sklave-Kitten." He nodded, confident in his naming. "Yep, Sklave-Kitten is right."

I felt as if I had been knighted. Getting a nickname in relation to my brothers? Being one of them? It's no exaggeration to say I'd been waiting my entire life for this moment.

"AK! Look who it is! Sklave-Kitten has arrived!" Todd shouted across the open lawn while jumping and pointing at me. A tall teenager walked toward us with a grin on his face and replied, "There she is! The third Sklaver!" He reached out his hand as if to shake mine before changing his mind and hugging me. "I've heard a lot about you."

He'd heard about me?! That was it, it was officially the best day of my life. It was both proof of my existence and a confirmation that my identity was inextricably linked to my siblings.

When you have spent your entire life (or if you're an older sibling, the vast majority) defining your identity in relation to another, then without that foil it can be hard to know if you even exist anymore. Older siblings become only children. Younger and middle siblings may suddenly become the oldest. Twins, no longer connected—are you even a twin anymore? New people you meet, friends you make—they don't know that other person ever existed.

For some, this feels like freedom, but the type of freedom that can be ridden with guilt.

For others, this feels like getting lost in a labyrinth with no David Bowie at the center.

It's as if your personal planetary orbit suddenly falls off-kilter and you begin to drift in space, disconnected from the universe that once encircled you. As one sibling put it, "My brother helped create my identity. As I've aged [since his death], my identity has always felt off."

For me, the question of "who am I if I'm not Ben and Sam's little sister?" was one of the most dizzying I've ever faced. My role as a younger sister always felt like the most sturdy, confident, well-secured element of my entire identity. Maybe I didn't know who I wanted to be when I grew up or what I wanted my future to look like, but I always knew I'd be a little sister.

When his older brother died by suicide, Stephen told me how his entire understanding of life went out the window. His big brother was his guidepost—even after he'd lost his job and struggled in his marriage, Stephen thought, "Okay, I shouldn't follow his lead on that specific thing; there's still a lot of these things that I will follow." But in his grief, Stephen found himself reassessing: "I had to have a reconciliation. If that didn't work, maybe all these things aren't right? Literally my entire world was upside down. There was a lot of internal examination around even my basic thought process."

It took me years before I could even begin to understand who I was if I wasn't Ben and Sam's sister. I wanted my identity to be associated with both of them—their vibrance and creativity. I didn't want to be "the girl with the dead brother," so I walked a line—talking about him less than I wanted but (seemingly) more often than I should. Never knowing what my life was without him in it before realizing, "I don't need to figure that out. I still have him. He still influenced who I am and how I engage with the world; death doesn't need to change that."

WHO WERE THEY?

There are also elements of your sibling's identity that may come out posthumously, and those can really mess with your head. In my research, sibling relationships impacted by significant mental health and addiction experienced this more frequently, as some did not know their sibling struggled with addiction or suicidal ideation. Especially for those who thought they had a close relationship, this revelation can be life-shattering. Why didn't they tell me? If I didn't know about this, what else didn't I know? Were we ever as close as I thought? These siblings often look back on their relationship through a new lens, trying to make sense of this perceived disconnect in the context of both their relationship and their identities.

RECENTERING

As the surviving sibling, we're left to recenter ourselves in an unfamiliar and often unwanted new world. When I faced this identity conundrum, the alarm bells went off in my head and I thought, "If I don't form an identity in this new world, then maybe I don't need to live in it! I will refuse this new world using brute force and an off-the-charts level of denial!" My inner child was screaming like a sitcom adolescent lashing out at a stepparent: "What could possibly go wrong?" Well, you know what went wrong: all of it. Life doesn't work that way. I couldn't will myself to remain in the safe, comfortable, familiar world that existed for the first twenty-five years of my life. Trust me, I tried.

A loss of this magnitude, regardless of the health and depth of your specific sibling relationship, has staggering effects on every element of our lives. It's unreasonable to expect that anyone could come out of it unchanged. Some changes will be for the better, others for the worse, but the change that happens is inevitable. At some point, if it hasn't happened yet, you'll have that moment of realization. Clouds will shift and the world will look different in the new light, and you'll realize that the future exists whether you like it or not—and you need to learn to engage with it. One sibling explained to me that after her older brother died of an overdose "I thought I could cling onto the person I was before it happened, and it took me about seven years to accept I needed help in my grief. I started therapy finally, and it has helped me so much. Now the biggest emotion left is just missing him so much. I don't think that ever goes away." The anger she felt has cleared, and the only emotion left is the painful evidence of their bond. Another sibling told me, with a hint of resignation in their voice, "I'm never going to be the same person I was, but I'm trying my best."

That's really all we can do, isn't it? Once we loosen the grip on the person we were before our loss, we can learn to take those first few steps toward creating ourselves in this new world.

YOUR WORST FEAR CAME TRUE. NOW WHAT?

Grief has a list of chronic side effects longer than a parody drug commercial:

- Dry eyes
- Insomnia
- Fatigue
- Rage
- Increased levels of cortisol and cortisol dysregulation
- Chronic headaches
- Nausea
- Lost sense of taste
- Confusion
- Increased cardiac risk
- Depression
- Panic attacks
- PTSD
- Ability to maintain a healthy perspective
- Resistance to sweating the small stuff
- Appreciation for life

Bet you didn't see those last few coming, right? I'm trying to keep you on your toes.

In taking a step back and observing themselves in the before times versus now, many siblings I spoke to were able to identify positive changes. I want to stress once again for my fellow guilt-ridden neurotics that acknowledging the good that has come from your loss does not mean you're okay with the loss, that it was "worth it," or that you'd ever have chosen this fate.

The perspective that comes with experiencing a loss as significant as ours can be a gift so powerful it will completely change how you engage and interact with the world. This new perspective on life came up time and time again in nearly all of my interviews, some referring to it as a "new superpower" and "sixth sense" that has helped them "grow into a better person." One study focusing on bereaved adolescent siblings also reported increased expressions of affection, greater purpose, and overall higher-than-average scores on a measure of self-concept.[1]

I think of it this way: My worst fear came true, and it was even worse than I expected. Now compare that to getting laid off, being rejected from your dream job, or getting dumped. In my experience, losing a job or partner is a terrible thing to happen and it can have a tremendous impact on your life, but it's not worse than losing my brother. So when that layoff comes, I honestly struggle to care because in my head I'm thinking, "As long as my family is safe and healthy, I don't care." And if I'm having a particularly spicy day, I think, "Go ahead and lay me off; just don't kill my family." That is not to say I don't still have my moments of stress and (more than a few) moments of anxiety—oh, I do—but deep down I know that I've dealt with worse, that I might not want to deal with this issue but I will survive it.

I went through a layoff in the course of writing this book, and more than a few colleagues asked how I was able to remain (mostly) calm through all of the chaos and instability. My perspective felt like a secret superpower, one that I didn't quite know how to express to my colleagues. After all, it's not as if I'd suggest it to others as a way to handle the current situation.

"Annie, how are you able to have such a great perspective on things?"

"Simple," I'd answer. "Lose a member of your immediate family, ideally a sibling, and you too can infuse your life with a healthy dose of perspective!"

But I'm realizing more and more that I can say that, though perhaps in a gentler way. Recently my best friend, who has known our family since she was born, told me that Ben's death has given her a new perspective as well. "I ask myself if this is really that bad—is it worse than losing Ben?" She shrugged. "So far the answer has always been no." I beamed. Not only because I'm glad that we both have this new perspective, but because her admission told me that she thinks about Ben—that he is a present and grounding force in her life, and that he continues to live on even outside our immediate family.

That said, you may read all that about perspective and yell out, "That's hogwash, Annie!" And in this moment, it might be for you. One sibling I spoke to described losing their sibling as "an ongoing experience," and wowwee is it ever. We are continuously learning more about ourselves and how we operate within the context of this new world. We are constantly forming and reforming our own identities, ones that were at once forged in the context of our sibling's presence and then again in the context of their absence. The loss is one we will carry for our entire lives. It doesn't need to define us, but it will be one key ingredient in our identity.

In a 2013 essay for the *New Yorker* titled "Now We Are Five," author David Sedaris explores this new dynamic following the death of his sister Tiffany. Sedaris is one of six siblings, and while the rest maintain a close relationship, he and Tiffany hadn't spoken in eight years. Even though they'd been estranged, the loss rocked his identity as he notes, "A person expects his parents to die. But a sibling? I felt I'd lost the identity I'd enjoyed since 1968, when my younger brother was born."[2]

In all my research, this struggle of identity development was a common thread, though I would argue that personal identity development is top of mind for most humans. The difference for bereaved siblings is that most do not *want* this to define them—they wanted to create their own identities without their sibling stepping in and stealing the show (yet again). As we discussed in Chapter 2, siblings are our touchstones to identity development, and it is natural for siblings to forge their identity both in relation to and in opposition to their sibling—with plentiful emphasis on the ways in which we're different from them. But without that comparison, how do we define ourselves? Does the touchstone remain, or does it disappear after death? I think that is entirely up to you.

In the years following the death of a sibling, the act of forming and reforming our identities can be imagined as a pendulum that may have some pretty significant swings before it settles anywhere.

That first wide swing is the act of absorbing and adjusting to our new world. It will continue to swing until we learn to carry the loss without denying or being defined by it, at which point (hopefully) we can settle into our own individual equilibriums. It won't happen quickly, and the swings will continue, but they lose some of their initial velocity.

THE PENDULUM. REDUX

Me Without You

These are those initial weeks, months, or years of acute grief. Not knowing how to answer when someone asked if you had siblings, the first time you used the past tense when referring to them, the day you became older than they'd ever be. This side of the pendulum is what we've been exploring thus far, and it's the side we're trying to emerge from.

Me as You

In addition to the erasure or reconfiguration of birth order we discussed in Chapter 5, there can be pressure from family (or from ourselves) to *become* the sibling who died or achieve their dreams in their absence. This treatment is especially common in siblings who experience loss at a younger age as their lives and identities are still forming. These expectations are unrealistic, unsatisfying, and developmentally harmful; but they exist.

Andrew is the youngest of three who lost both of his older brothers within ten years of each other. After the loss of his second brother, he explained, "I was treated like an only child, which really hurt. For some reason people just expected me to be okay and to suddenly be perfect." When I asked Andrew what he'd tell himself if he could go back in time to those first few weeks after his brother died, he replied, "I'd tell myself that my feelings are valid. That I will always be a sibling even though they are gone. That I don't have to be perfect as the only living child."

Ryan's brother had a sometimes-tense relationship with their father, and as a result she believes her father carries a tremendous amount of guilt. Her relationship with their father had been her own, with their own unique love and challenges, but in the aftermath of her brother's death, she's found herself the recipient of her father's attempts to make amends. It didn't matter that the issues he's trying to resolve had nothing to do with her; she has effectively been put in the role of stand-in for her brother.

The pressure to assume your sibling's identity doesn't always come from external sources. It is just as common for siblings to forge this role for themselves, often starting as an act of respect or tribute. I came very close to falling into this trap myself, and frankly I'm not exactly sure how I avoided it. When my brother was killed, he left behind a small non-profit he had started after his first deployment to the Horn of Africa. His organization, ClearWater Initiative, built wells in northern Uganda. It was a small but mighty organization that had already completed multiple projects in the few short years between its inception and his death. I was in school for toy design at the time and often considered quitting to run ClearWater myself. No one asked me to; in fact, my parents had taken over daily operations and put zero pressure on Sam or me to be involved. The board was made up of Ben's friends and colleagues, all of whom had extensive experience in the world of NGOs, humanitarian aid, and non-profits. I had none of those things, but I still thought perhaps it was my path. After deciding to stay the course with my degree and career plans, I battled a tremendous amount of guilt. Was I being selfish? Did his work matter more than mine? What would happen to ClearWater without him? Was that going to die too?

I'm glad I didn't abandon my identity and take up Ben's. In hind-sight, it may have been one of the most sound decisions I made that first year. I would have had no clue what I was doing and, more importantly, I wouldn't have been happy there. Living someone else's dream isn't a virtuous tribute—in my case I think it would have been a cop-out. Ben had a clear idea of what he wanted, and I was a lost twenty-five-year-old. Taking up his dreams would have been the easy way out. Finding my own path would be much more difficult.

There are, of course, instances in which one sibling may have taken on the role of the deceased—whether in life or in work—and it was fulfilling and valuable. I'm not suggesting that it can't work, but it can only work if it is what you genuinely want and there is no resentment for being put in that position. Kat explained that she became a therapist because "I've always been that person" beginning as a child when she had to help her brother. Did she resent that? "I've learned that we all have a lot less control than we think," she explained. "I know that I'm not responsible for other people's emotions even though that was the role I was put in." Her experience is what inspired her to do the work she does, but it's on her terms.

Losing a sibling does not mean you need to live for both of you; it means you need to live for yourself more than ever before.

Me and You

The pendulum's resting place is the sweet spot where we learn to live our own lives with as much (or as little) of our sibling's presence as we choose, in whatever ways we choose. The key here being choice, specifically your choice—no one else's. This is the act of learning to carry the loss with us. The pendulum will still swing from time to time, some swings bigger than others, but if we find equilibrium, we can always return to it.

Dan's brother was killed in combat, and Dan strives to "live a life worthy of his sacrifice." This does not mean Dan joined the army or took up his brother's causes—it means he lives every day with honesty, integrity, and an appreciation for life.

Sarah pursued her PhD in substance abuse in education as a tool to learn and understand what her brother was struggling with. She told me that she "had to do it for my healing," and it did just that—it helped her heal. Now she works as a school psychiatrist where "there are pieces of him in all that I do." Sarah found purpose and passion through her brother's struggles with addiction and death—that's different than living *for* him. This is a way she is able to live *with* him ever-present.

Devin recounted the moment when he realized "my improvement of my own soul is my connection with my brother, and that remains. He was proud of me in my life when I didn't really apply myself. And now from the other side he can really take pleasure and joy and pride in me being the best version of myself. I can become king in my own way."

thirteen

Looking for Signs

I want you to reach me / and show me all the things no one
else can see / so what you feel becomes mine as well.

—Blues Traveler

I used to have a hard time believing in things I could not see. After Ben
was killed, we were given strict instructions by the army not to open
the casket. As Jews, we don't do open caskets in general, but this meant
we could not identify the body. How was I supposed to know that it was
Ben in that box and not some other soldier? What if it was empty? What
if Ben was a prisoner of war or had run off into the hills of Afghanistan?

The inability to see the body of the deceased is known to hinder a
mourner's ability to find closure. This is not distinct to siblings, but due
to the societal diminishment of the relationship, siblings are often told,
rather than shown, evidence of their loss. In their absence, grieving siblings will actively seek signs from their brothers and sisters and exhibit

distress without them. "I'm moving homes tomorrow and I've got so much anxiety over it," Margie told me. Her brother had been gone seven years at this point, yet she was in a panic: "Will he know my new address? How will he know where to visit me? I need him to come visit me in my dreams."

As time passed after Ben's death, I became increasingly desperate to feel his presence. To feel any tangible proof of his continued existence in my universe. That's when my friend Beth, who had also lost her older brother, encouraged me to look for signs. "I don't believe in signs," I told her. "I wouldn't even know where to start." "Ask for something very specific," she instructed. "Something you don't see every day, something like a blue flower."

So that's what I did. Because I was completely incapable of being creative, I asked Ben to show me blue flowers. A week later, on my way to work, I noticed a large patch of blue flowers and wrote it off immediately. I'm sure they'd been there previously; I just hadn't noticed. That was evidence of the power of suggestion, not the existence of signs. The next day I saw my psychiatrist, an older woman with a thick New York accent whose clothes hadn't been particularly memorable in the past. That day she wore a blouse covered in blue flowers, blue pants, and Doc Marten–style boots with blue flowers embroidered on them.

There he was, making sure I saw him without a shadow of a doubt.

There's a scene in *The Man with Two Brains* in which Steve Martin asks his dead wife to send him a sign. The lights flicker, furniture flies around the room, her portrait spins on the wall, and a voice from beyond starts howling. When it all dies down, Steve Martin says, "Any kind of sign; I'll keep on the lookout for it." I've seen that movie a dozen times, but until I laid eyes on those blue flower boots, I'd never realized how many portraits Ben had been spinning right in front of my eyes.

GREAT, I'M A FEELER

A few weeks later I stood on a street corner wondering how the hell Beth had talked me into spending $300 on this. I did not believe in mediums.

I did not believe in psychics or supernatural things. Sure, I'd had some weird things happen recently that could be considered "signs," and yes, maybe I'd been afraid to go to a medium before because I *did* believe, and maybe that was the scary part.

So here I was, going to see a medium. They buzzed me into the building, and as I cautiously walked inside their apartment, the smell of homemade chicken soup and incense filled my senses and immediately calmed me down. I looked to my left at the galley kitchen and saw a big pot bubbling away with large chunks of onion, carrots, and celery floating among the chicken bones and aromatics.

"Oh, you're a feeler. Shit. You're a big feeler." I turned back to Gem, the medium, and they were eyeing me with a kind of nervous excitement: "Look, I have goosebumps and we haven't even started talking. You've got a lot with you; we better start early. Put your stuff down and let's go. You can't record this, but you can take notes, so grab your notebook and take a seat on the couch. I'll be there in a minute."

I had brought a new blank notebook for this. Yes, I did like any excuse to get a new notebook that I'd never actually fill, but in this case I just couldn't imagine writing down the details of this session in a notebook with anything else. What was I supposed to do, write messages from my dead brother transmitted through a medium in my work notebook?

Notebook in hand, I cautiously crossed the living room and took a seat at one end of the long couch. As Gem began to explain their gift and what I should expect from the session, I was overcome with emotion and fought back tears. They hadn't even said anything about me yet. Why was I ready to cry?

"I can't guarantee that we'll talk to your brother, or that anyone will come through. We do have free will after all, even on the other side."

I nodded. I knew this was a possibility; I wasn't even sure I believed hearing from Ben was real, but I was ready for this—whatever this was.

"I can see that there is a very raw loss, something recent and painful," they continued. "The pain is very new and raw for people in your family."

I cut them off. "It was ten years ago. It'll be ten years next month." I officially do not believe in mediums.

"Ten years? Oh, girl, why didn't you come see me earlier? Okay, ten years. Well, you all are acting like it just happened. You're stuck. People in your family are stuck."

I nod. They're right; we are stuck—some of us more than others. I know none of us *want* to move forward; we don't want to move into a world without him in it. We've found a new normal, but we haven't moved forward, not really. Maybe this medium was on to something.

"He wasn't alone. Not for a second. He's here and he wants you to know that. That's the most important thing you need to know right now. Your mom is worried that he's alone, but he wasn't—not for a second. He wants you to tell her that. And he never felt any pain; she needs to know that too."

The tears come now, overflowing from me in breathless sobs. I nod silently, unable to form any words, as they hand me a box of tissues.

"From all my experience talking with souls on the other side, I can tell you that he's telling the truth; he didn't feel anything. Our souls leave our bodies moments before we die so we do not feel anything. Let me ask you, did he have a breathing tube?"

"No," I manage to get out in a whisper.

"There's something right here," they said, pointing to a spot at the base of their neck between their collar bone. "Something here is burning like it's on fire."

"I . . . I don't know. He never had a breathing tube." I absently put my hand on my chest where they'd been pointing and felt something on myself. My locket. I reached under my shirt and pulled it out so they could see it. "Is it this?"

"What's in the locket?"

I carefully open the locket. "His picture."

"Well, there you go." They continue but I'm still clutching the locket in shock. "Whose name starts with a Z? Someone with a Z was waiting for him when his soul left his body."

"My Grandma Zelma, she died a few years before him."

"He says that's it; she was waiting for him and the big guy was right behind her with a joke."

I laugh in disbelief. My Grandpa Archie was a very large man who used to call our house when he knew we were at school and leave jokes on our answering machine. He'd deliver the setup and then wait in silence for a few seconds before blurting out the punchline and giggling. Grandpa was there. They were both there. This was real. "When we pass there's always someone waiting for us; we're never alone. Grandma was the first person he saw, and he'll be waiting for you. He will be the first person you see, but it won't be for a long time."

"He wouldn't have done anything differently," they continued. "He says you need to know that. He wouldn't have done a single thing differently. He knows it's harder for you here without him and for that he is sorry, but he'd still do it all the same." Gem takes a sip of their tea and looks at me quizzically. "Are you a journalist?"

"No." I shake my head and furrow my brow, confused.

"He's talking about an interview; he said you did an interview this morning."

"Oh my god. I . . . this morning I interviewed his best friend. I'm trying to capture his story, and I'm starting with kind of an oral history. Today was my first interview. How did you know that? How did he know that?"

"YESSSS! That's it! Oh, he is jazzed about this. He knows because you're doing it together, he's doing this project with you. You need to let it evolve. It starts with writing but it's going to be a film—don't hire one of your friends to do the music. The music is going to be very important; don't farm it out to a friend, you need a professional."

"Wait, is this you talking or Ben?"

"It's Ben, I don't give a fuck who does the music. He says he's going to lead you; you're collaborating on this. You're not alone. He's been here the whole time and now he's going to show you. Don't overthink this and don't overcomplicate it, okay? You need to tell him okay."

"Okay," I say, stunned. "Okay, we're doing it together."

"Oh man, you're going to laugh one day when you look back at this and thought you didn't have a purpose. You can stop looking for purpose now; it's right here. This is it. This is your platform. Ever since you were a kid you've been telling stories; you've always wanted to tell the stories of injustice, and this is your first step. His will be the first of many stories you tell."

SIGN, SIGN, EVERYWHERE A SIGN

Turns out, I wasn't the only one looking for signs from their sibling—not by a long shot. Devin looked for the same after his brother's passing and sees them everywhere; he described his brother's presence as "an invisible hand." It's that supporting hand to help you up, wave hello, give you a high five, flick you on the nose, and remind you that their presence remains.

Once I was open to feeling that kind of presence, I saw (or heard) it everywhere, most often in the form of music. Sometimes the songs are a reminder of his love, and sometimes they're the obvious weapon of an older brother determined to mess with his little sister. My son goes through phases in which he listens to the same song on repeat. One such phase, much to my husband and my chagrin, was an obsession with Journey's "Don't Stop Believing." As we got into the car one Sunday morning, Archie requested his song and Aaron and I both refused. We couldn't listen to it one more time, we desperately needed a break. "We're listening to the radio," Aaron declared. "We're not taking requests." He turned on a local radio station and I bet you can guess what song came through the speakers . . .

Just a small-town girl.

Livin' in a lonely world.

Archie squealed in delight as Aaron and I looked at each other and whispered, "Very funny, Ben." I swear I could hear his giggle from beyond the grave as that invisible hand gave his nephew a high five.

I've decided to stop thinking so much about the physics and legitimacy of the signs because regardless of their origin, they make me smile. Maybe that song coming on was pure coincidence, but whatever it was it reminded me of my brother and the goofy uncle he would have been, and I like that feeling. It reminds me that Ben was real, and he still is. I've decided I don't need to know how the sausage is made, you know? Magic tricks lose their magic once you know how they're done, and I want these moments to remain magical.

In the course of writing this book there was a super blood moon lunar eclipse. It was during a time in the pandemic when we were all deeply desperate for good (or at least not harrowing) news, so the eclipse was a big deal. I'd been exploring my woo-woo side, so I channeled my energy into the moon too.

I made a crystal grid (first I learned what a crystal grid was, then I made one).

I set my intentions.

I read about the supermoon.

But I never saw the super blood moon lunar eclipse.

It rained that night. The sky was so full of clouds that there wasn't a sliver of moon in sight—which is saying a lot because apparently there was a great deal of moon to be seen.

But here's the magical thing . . . I didn't care.

I knew that the eclipse was happening, whether I saw it or not. That's kind of the whole point, right? The eclipse is not dependent on you seeing it. It does not need your eyewitness account to validate its existence. You do not need to see it in order to feel its power.

Learning to feel Ben's presence, to know that he will continue to exist in the ether whether I see him or not, has been life-changing. Trusting in the power of our relationship to be eternal gives pieces of him back to me. The relationship doesn't look like I ever expected it to be, but I know it's there whether I see it or not.

CONTINUING BONDS

This type of connection is called "continuing bonds" and is one way in which we form ongoing attachments with the deceased. This theory, introduced in 1996, is widely accepted by psychiatrists and grief experts alike and builds on the notion that grief is the expression of continued love and is not something we "get over" but rather something we carry with us. You may be skeptical, or perhaps you don't want to continue this relationship, and that's okay. Continuing bonds are not always a good thing—we'll get to that soon.

In a 2003 study on bereaved adolescent siblings, researchers found that the most essential element of the bereaved person's grief processing was that they engaged in a search for meaning that included the development of continuing bonds.[1] These bonds helped the bereaved move forward in their new world, with a new feeling of sibling camaraderie and connection. Now, these bonds are not something that happens immediately, or something that can be forced. Continuing bonds develop over time, as this study noted that the process took years and for some siblings remains ongoing. One beautiful thing this study showed was that for adolescents these bonds shift and change at each new developmental phase. Why is that beautiful? Because it means the relationship is alive, and like all personal relationships, it can grow and change *with* us. It's beautiful because I hear the voices of all the siblings I spoke to who expressed regret and remorse for not trying hard enough to have a relationship with their sibling in life, always assuming there would be more time and a shared adulthood, and I think, "Maybe it's not too late."

If you are looking to discover and nurture continuing bonds with your sibling, there are a few things you can do to help kick-start the process:

1. Talk to them. I'm not kidding. Close your eyes and imagine they're in front of you, then start talking.
2. Talk to other people about them (more on that in the next chapter!)—especially people who never knew them.
3. Explore an interest or hobby they were passionate about. Never understood why your brother liked CrossFit so much? Go to a class and see for yourself.
4. Look at pictures of them. Hang their photo on the wall and think of them each time you catch sight of it. Don't hide them away.

5. Consider embodying their values or lessons they taught you and live a life they'd be proud of.
6. Create your own rituals and traditions and stick to them as long as they're still serving you.

The highlight of many of my interviews were these stories of continuing bonds. These were the moments when we would smile, the dark clouds that had loomed overhead would often part, and there might even be (gasp) laughter. In the next chapter we'll focus more deeply on why telling these stories is so important, but first I want to give some of these siblings the opportunity to tell you about their moments of continued connection and presence—in their own words.

KENNY'S STORY

My brother Kyle had a close friend who he worked with at a termite company, and it turned out that the friend's wife was my sister's Sunday school teacher. Now, about two years after Kyle died my wife and I moved into a new house, and we threw a birthday party for my sister at the house and she invited them—Kyle's friend and the son and his wife. When they pulled into the neighborhood, Kyle's friend tells his wife, "Me and Kyle did a house in this neighborhood." He's looking around and says, "I actually trained Kyle at a house in this neighborhood." So she asks him which house and he says, "It's the yellow one, all the way in the back." So they come around the corner and he says, "This is it, this is the house right here." And his wife says, "That's Kenny and Megan's house."

They tell me this and I realize Kyle has been in this house, and we didn't buy it for two years after he died. I'm sitting there thinking, "Was this real? Kyle's been in this house." On top of that, the way we got the house was . . . well . . . it kind of just fell in our lap. We'd wondered how we were able to get this house the way we did, and then I know. I know how we got the house now.

I don't know how to word it . . . joy I guess is a good term. We were supposed to get this house because he was in it. He was in here and his friend was able to tell us stories about Kyle being in this house. It makes you feel good knowing that even though he isn't here, he was here; even before I was, he was here.

DEVIN'S STORY

There are certain events that transpire only my brother Barron could create. I had his rollerblades and they meant everything to me; they were *his* rollerblades. We used to rollerblade all the time; roller hockey was, like, one of the top three things we did together. After he died, I was staying with my friend Hans in this beautiful neighborhood and I'm rollerblading. I would ride every day and leave them outside. One morning I went outside and they weren't there; I lost it. You try to hold on to everything that was irreplaceable, you know? Hans was out of town, he's not even there, but I asked him a bunch of questions like did he put them away? I am really freaking out. I can usually keep my composure, but I was not then, not at all. My blood is boiling, and I keep thinking to myself, "How could someone do that? How could someone come into *my* grief, up in *my* house, and take Barron's rollerblades that meant the world to me?"

After a day of that I said, "Fuck it, I have to get my own rollerblades." Of course I find one pair of the ones I want in Toronto, Canada. The best rollerblades I've ever owned. As I freaking put those on, I gotta tell you, it was so obvious that Barron's saying, "Dude, you're bugging. I stole those motherfuckers because you can't keep using those old things; you need to have your own blades, man, those were old fucking blades. You want to be a king, have the best pair of rollerblades for yourself. This is your time to upgrade." When they arrived, there was a leaf on the package, which I still possess because leaves were our whole thing. The leaf was on top of the package like a bow.

He's so alive. Now he's just flying around the universe like a bright white light. I can feel when he says, "What's up?" and I can feel when he visits. That connection is only getting stronger over time.

STEPHEN'S STORY

There are songs that remind me of my brother; one is a song called "Green Grass and High Tides" by the Outlaws, which was a country rock band from the '70s. He used to refer to it as the "first song in the car song," as in, when you get in the car that's the song you put on first. So now a year or two after he died, I had to go to New York for a work trip, and I was going to see my sister-in-law (his widow) and my niece and my nephew. I turn on the car, I back out of my driveway, and I'm not even to the end of my street when this song comes on. It's an eight-minute song—it's not often played on the radio. My first thought was "What the fuck? There's no way." I took a picture of it and sent it to my sister, telling her, "I just got in the car and this came on the radio." Sure enough, she responded, "Oh my god, that's the first song in this car song."

When stuff like that happens, I think, that is not a coincidence.

WHEN THE BONDS SHOULD BREAK

Just as we need to leave space for the possibility that there are no good memories and deeply flawed relationships, so too must we acknowledge that not every bond should be continued. Continued bonds are not a magical one-size-fits-all cure to grief; there's no sisterhood of the traveling bereaved pants. The same research that found continuing bonds to be a positive tool for living with grief also noted that "in instances where the relationship between the siblings was primarily ambivalent or conflictual, the connection to their deceased siblings may be disturbing or even frightening."[2] When the loss carries feelings of guilt, regret, or conflict, the feeling of connection and continued bonds may be no comfort at all.

For these reasons, continuing bonds can be as unique as our individual grieving styles, and it's equally important to respect whatever style feels right for you. If fostering continuing bonds is something that feels comforting or healing for you, then there are things we can do to help you get there. But if you don't, if these bonds bring more stress than peace, then please do not forge them. Relief might be stigmatized in grief (go back to Chapter 7 if you need a refresher), but that doesn't mean it isn't real. Your life might be better off without that relationship, and your grief might be more about the absence of a healthy sibling relationship than about your actual sibling. Try not to confuse the two.

TRANSITIONAL OBJECTS

When my kids were babies, our pediatrician recommended introducing a "transitional object"—something that is associated with us (our smells, etc.) that the baby could keep with them even when we weren't around. She explained that it could make the transition to day care and babysitters a bit easier since the baby would still have a physical reminder of us in their new environment. Turns out babies aren't the only ones who need transitional objects.

Physical belongings become the transitional objects we cling to as we move from the life we've known to one that feels more dangerous and uncertain. Multiple studies have found that it was helpful for mourners to have or wear possessions that belonged to the deceased as a physical reminder of their existence and continued presence. This is no different for siblings. Just as the existence of these objects brings many siblings a sense of comfort, those who did not possess such objects noted a sense of despair that they had no physical expression of the deceased.

The objects I've been attached to have changed over the years. These days Ben's diaries are among my most prized possessions, but there were those first nine years after his death when I never even picked them up. Instead, I found myself clinging to photos of him and the letters and emails we'd exchanged, wanting to remember and re-remember every moment together for fear of losing them. I suppose I had less interest in the time we were apart; I needed my transitional objects to contain traces of both of us to prove that we once existed together.

WHEN THE BONDS ARE STRONGER AFTER DEATH

For some siblings I spoke to, especially those whose sibling suffered physical or mental illness, the relationship forged through continuing bonds can feel even more real than the relationship they had on earth. Devin's brother was sick for so long, it was like his body was holding his spirit hostage, and he told me, "In a way he's more alive because he doesn't have to suffer." For those who suffered addiction, siblings noted that there was no longer pressure to "fix" things or save them; that energy was now free to focus more on the person, imperfections and all. Kat experienced sibling rivalry with her brother while he was alive, but after his death she felt a significant shift in their relationship dynamic. Rather than the rivalry she'd known so well, she now feels a deep sense of loyalty and a desire to defend him and his legacy. For Molly, the void that came along with her brother's death was the thing that drove her to understand their relationship in the first place—what must they have shared for her to feel such deep loss now?

For years after the 2014 release of the film *Boyhood*, and at seemingly random times, the song that presided over the film's trailer and soundtrack would pop into my head. For a few days I'd find myself listening to it on repeat, as it captured that magical balance of sadness and wonder. This was before I had really processed my own loss. Time had passed but my grief still felt fresh, and I was clinging to whatever scraps of Ben I still had. I was focused so much on what was lost, desperate to find recordings of his voice for fear I'd forget it, and him. I was still fighting against the new world and unable to see any way in which my relationship with him could go beyond what it last had been.

Time passed. More time passed. I had a lot of therapy, did a lot of processing, started feeling his presence fill that void again, and started writing this book. I hadn't heard the song in years and for whatever reason that familiar tug started again, and I went back to it: "Hero" by Family of the Year. The opening lines that once haunted me for reasons I couldn't understand rang out, and this time they hit differently.

Let me go / I don't wanna be your hero.

I listened again and again and again, each time feeling a pang of anguish at the opening plea to "let me go." I didn't want to let him go; I'd clung to him for so long. But I don't think the boy in the song is asking to be let go completely; he wants to be freed of expectation and pressure.

He wants permission to be flawed, to walk with everyone else. Ben didn't want to be untouchable on some pedestal; the guy's signature big-brother move was to tell me about all the ways he'd messed up. He wants to be the prankster uncle who teaches his nieces and nephew how to properly annoy their parents and supplies them with unlimited fireworks, not the war hero frozen in time.

The biggest gift that came from developing continuing bonds, for me, is that it has given me back a very present and evolving relationship with my brother. He's no longer frozen or high up on that pedestal, and once again we're aging together, just in a different way. I also give myself a lot more freedom to imagine what he would be like if he hadn't died, and you know what? It's kind of fun. For example, at thirty-two his hairline was noticeably receding, and my little sister adrenaline spikes at the knowledge (not assumption, *knowledge*) that he would be bald by now. Gah, it makes me so happy to imagine bald Ben.

fourteen

Telling Our Story

Truth is just like time, it catches up and it just keeps going.

—Dar Williams

I was really excited to write this chapter. I know "excited" is an unexpected way to describe writing a book about grief, but this chapter . . . this chapter is magic because our stories are magic. Storytelling is what has kept us alive for generation after generation. It's how we were able to thrive and evolve and know which berries poisoned that last guy. But it's not only about physical survival. You see, when you start telling a first-person narrative, something truly remarkable happens: the listener's brain waves sync up with those of the narrator. The listener's brain waves *actually change*, in a measurable way, to align with those of the narrator. Stories don't just teach us which berries are poisonous. They teach us empathy and train our brains to think differently. This phenomenon is called neural coupling, and it allows us to rapidly form relationships and build empathy.

Empathy, in this case, is not a theoretical feeling. When we listen to a story that holds our attention and transports us to the narrator's world, our brains release oxytocin. Oxytocin is the same chemical released in our brains after childbirth and is essential to human bonding, which is why some researchers call it the love hormone and others the empathy hormone. Studies of oxytocin and its effects on the brain have proven that "when the brain synthesizes oxytocin, people are more trustworthy, generous, charitable, and compassionate. . . . What we know is that oxytocin makes us more sensitive to social cues around us."[1] Stories are what bond us together. They are what allow us to find community and support from people who didn't experience our same loss but who can empathize with it. It's also why hearing stories of other people's experiences can resonate so strongly in our minds, helping us feel less alone and normalizing grief's unpredictable impact.

Margie wished more people had asked for those stories, had allowed her to open up about them. In fact, it's the biggest piece of advice she'd give someone who is supporting a grieving sibling: "Ask about their sibling. Let them tell you all the stories about them. Say their sibling's name." In my conversations with other grieving siblings, I always ask them what they'd want to say to their past selves in the throes of grief, and a common theme emerged—talk about them:

"I'd tell myself that whatever you're feeling right now is valid and okay. You will always be a sibling even though they are gone. You don't have to justify your grief to anyone. That you're not alone."

"Don't be afraid to tell people about your sibling and what happened to them. Talk to a counselor or therapist. Don't keep it all balled up inside."

"Talk about what happened. Don't be ashamed or afraid of what people will say. They won't judge you or think you're weak. Sharing your feelings will empower you. Talk about what you're feeling. Find a creative outlet and put the pain into that."

"It took more than ten years before I began to really process my sister's death. The sadness and sense of loss is not something that is easily quantifiable, but it really doesn't go away either. I think the sooner a person begins to grieve and work through the loss, the better off they will be."

Just because you've buried your sibling's body does not mean you have to bury their spirit, their memories, or their love. They are alive in your stories.

STORIES HELP REDEFINE US

When siblings shared stories with me, they lit up. There were smiles, jokes, and genuine laughs. It was obvious that sharing the stories of their siblings' lives was, in many ways, a relief. While many people had resisted the urge to tell these stories for fear of alienation or discomfort, they had been simmering under the surface just itching to get out. I love telling people all the weird things Ben would do; I love poking fun at him and making him human again. That's what stories do: they make us human.

Telling stories isn't only about keeping your loved one's memory alive. In many ways that is secondary to the true virtue of stories. Stories are what shape and define our identity. After a traumatic event, like the loss of a sibling, we're left reshaping our identities (you know that from Chapters 5 and 12), and stories are how we do it. There are a lot of external factors that go into identity creation, many of which we have no control over, but we do have control over our own actions—how we respond, how we process, how we grow. That is the story. The story isn't what happened *to* us, that's just the context. The story is all the ways we respond to those factors, how we make meaning of it all, and what we choose to do next.

When attempting to process a new experience, there are two main paths: assimilative processing or accommodative processing. Assimilative processing happens when we absorb the experience or event into our existing story. In that way, the event melts in with all the other events that have happened in our lives. Accommodative processing, on the other hand, requires us to revise our story, to change the narrative in order to make sense of the experience. Research indicates that taking the time and doing the hard work that accommodative processing requires has some significant benefits, including an increased sense of meaning and purpose and positive mental health.

LOSS ISN'T YOUR ONLY STORY

You are the author, editor, publisher, producer, director, and main character in your own story. In *The Healing Power of Storytelling*, Dr. Annie Brewster explains, "We make meaning out of what happens to us, reflected in the stories we tell about ourselves, and in doing so, we get to choose how we move forward. While life is full of events we do not expect and cannot control, we play an active role in determining how the story unfolds by the moments we choose to remember and how we choose to remember them."[2]

One of our stories is that of our loss, of course, and it's an important story to tell. But that is by no means the only story. For most of us the stories of life greatly outnumber the stories of loss, and those are the stories that lay the path to immortality. What if we talked about life? What if instead of avoiding any sibling talk, we focused on telling the stories that make us smile and remind us how beautiful life can be?

Telling these stories does not make you self-absorbed. It does not make you needy or attention-seeking or any of those other negative things we tell ourselves. Telling stories of our siblings and our loss is essential for the processing of grief and making sense of what the hell happened. When I spoke with Dr. Danielle Busby, licensed clinical psychologist and cofounder of Black Mental Wellness, she explained this as a healthy and productive way to process the loss, using stories as a tool to understand how we want to move forward, remember, and honor our loved ones. The more you tell your story, the more comfortable you will become in it, and witnessing these stories will help dissipate the pain. A study from the University of Missouri showed that providing the mourner an opportunity to tell and retell their story actually reduces symptoms of complicated grieving.[3]

YOU ARE NOT THE SOLE KEEPER

There are two reasons why I use the social media app TikTok. The first is to watch funny dog videos with my kids, and the second is to follow @manicpixiemom. Each of her videos follows the same formula: a time-lapse video of her cleaning old gravestones while telling the stories of those buried there. Some of these graves are over a century old, and while the stone may weather and age the stories somehow remain. Of course, this isn't true of all graves, and many remain unmarked and unknown, but the stories we do have allow these people to be revived and live on. Their stories live in me now, along with 2.7 million other followers.

The mere existence of stories brings us one step closer to immortality. I never met my great-grandmother, a chicken farmer, but I know that she insisted all her daughters go to college in the 1920s and '30s. My children never met their Uncle Ben, but they can tell you all about him—that his favorite food was pumpkin pie, he had a dog named Juno, and he loved fireworks on the beach. Those pieces of him live on, his presence still felt in those moments. Now that I've shared those stories with them, he will live on without me. My son can have pumpkin pie at a friend's house and smile remembering the stories he's heard about the lengths his uncle would go to for a slice of pie. I've shared a small piece of the load, the web has grown larger, and there is a little bit more Ben in the world.

Think about all the people you've never met but know way too much about.

I know the name of the kid who punched David Bowie in the eye, resulting in his mismatched pupils and appearance of having two differently colored eyes. *Why do I know that?* Because for a few years my son's favorite book was David Bowie's life story.

I know that Stephen Colbert's mom would practice fainting in her kitchen and taught her eleven children the key to a convincing faint. *Why do I know that?* Because he talked about it on his show after she passed away.

I know that Iestyn's brother loved *Star Wars*, and the two of them loved building LEGOs together as children. *Why do I know that?* Because he told me. And from now on, I'll think of them when I see *Star Wars* paraphernalia or witness my children playing LEGOs together (and so will you).

As one sibling told me, "As long as we keep speaking his name, he'll be immortal." Another noted, "Talking about her and acting on her behalf keeps her around."

One of the first questions I asked in my interviews was the name of their deceased siblings. I'd write it on a little index card and keep it just offscreen, terrified I'd forget or mispronounce it throughout the interview. Sure, I could have referred to them more anonymously as "brother" or "sister," but there was something very special that happened when their name was said—a split second of joy. The first time they said the name, most siblings said it with a smile and their shoulders would relax. Throughout the conversation, using their name allowed us to talk about them personally, and many noted that it felt good to say their name out loud with a new person.

After telling me stories about his sister, Robert reflected, "I love knowing someone else is thinking about her." The knowledge that you're not alone in your grief or the sole caretaker of their memory is so empowering. You've allowed them to continue to exist in your world.

Even if you did not participate in my specific interviews, you still have an opportunity each and every day to feel your sibling's presence and immortality if it brings you joy. In speaking with people who knew your sibling, you have the opportunity to learn new things about them and add to your memory bank. Siblings report that these conversations leave them feeling validated, connected to both their sibling and the storyteller, and comforted knowing they're not alone.

THE HARDEST STORIES OF ALL

Okay, so telling these stories is a key to resilient grief processing, continuing bonds, and (dare I say) our overall happiness. That's great. You know what else is good for us? Avoiding processed food, sleeping at least eight hours a night, and drinking tons of water; just because it's good for us doesn't make it easy.

The first time I wrote about the events of Ben's death, of the moment I heard the news and the surreal forty-eight hours that followed, was when I was writing the proposal for this very book. I know what Ben would have said. He would have told me to write it down that night, the next day, the next week . . . he would have told me to write it all down—the emotions, the struggles, the tears. He would have told me to write down our memories, preserve them on the pages. But I didn't, I couldn't. As we've already covered, the idea that I should do something "because Ben would have wanted that" was not a compelling reason for me to do anything.

Stephanie Wittels Wachs *did* immediately begin to write about the death of her brother Harris, and her book *Everything Is Horrible and Wonderful* includes those stories chronicling the first year after his death. When I spoke to Stephanie, one of my first questions was simply "How?"

"I didn't set out to write a book," she explained, "it just started as notes on my phone. I process things through creativity, so that's what I did. My only goal was waking up every day."

I suppose that's a core difference between us. Stephanie knew that writing would help, that it was a process to heal, and it was done with the intention of doing just that. No more. No less. I was afraid to write; I didn't see writing as a way to process, I saw it as a way to finalize. It's the difference between writing with a pencil and writing with a Sharpie.

So I didn't write. Instead, I thought about writing and obsessed over it in my head for ten years. I was afraid that writing it down would make it all real—the loss, the pain, the sadness. If it existed on the page, then I couldn't run from it.

What I've found is quite the opposite. Telling these stories, talking about Ben—it doesn't somehow make him *more* dead; he can't be more dead. Instead, talking about him is slowly bringing him back to life. Just as we all grieve differently, we'll all find a different type of comfort in the stories. Some of you will be ready to talk before others, but when you're ready, your stories will become an integral part of their legacy and your healing.

Telling these stories isn't always easy, and the biggest hurdles siblings report fall into two buckets: language and audience.

Language

Tenses, emotions, projections, nuance—so much is wrapped up in the words we choose to use when we tell our stories. These aren't choices that can be easily made based on rules of grammar or traditional storytelling because these are loaded emotional decisions. Do I talk about my brother in the past or present tense? He's gone, but he's still very present. Which are his stories and which are mine? Am I allowed to tell his stories since he isn't around to tell them? But what if I get something wrong? What if I misrepresent him and he isn't here to set the record straight? And why do we even have tenses? Why are tenses so hard?

Take a deep breath.

Now get out of your head.

What tense should you use? Whatever tense feels right in that moment.

What if they can't set the record straight? As long as you're telling your story, it's okay. Don't presume to know anything you don't actually know; be honest with the holes and gaps in the story, but tell the story. They'll forgive you if you get a few things wrong.

The language doesn't get any easier for people who are otherwise comfortable writing. In fact, it can be more challenging to tell these stories when telling stories is something you're otherwise an expert at. One sibling told me, "I fancy myself a writer and I can't seem to write much about how this loss feels. It's something that's beyond language."

I think the real language barrier, if we're being honest with each other here (which we are), is that the death of a sibling can throw reality into question. More so than others, siblings impacted by suicide and addiction report that they're left questioning their own memories; what was real and what was hiding under the surface. Unfortunately, there's no easy way to confirm or reenact those memories with this new perspective, and the result can be a very disorienting lens through which some struggle to see. I will never know how much information Ben hid from us. Did he know how dangerous his role was and downplay it when talking to family? Did he believe he was telling us the truth, or protecting us?

I will never know, but there are some things I *do* know:

- I know he loved me.
- I know he made sure I felt his love and support.
- I know he liked tapered jeans, though I'll never understand why.
- I know in high school he'd pack three PB&J sandwiches to supplement the school's hot lunch because otherwise it simply wasn't enough food.
- I know he believed in the importance of the work he was doing.
- I know he often took our mom's side when I was mad at her, that bastard.
- I know he bought me a plane ticket to visit him when I had my heart broken.

Those are the stories I can tell. Stories about how he made me feel, laugh, scream, grow. Telling stories doesn't mean telling *every* story, maybe it means telling (and retelling) the one story that makes you smile, or the story that is hard to tell but essential to hear. These are your stories, and you get to decide which stories are told.

Stories exist beyond the spoken word, and sometimes those are the easiest to start with—before the words have formed. Stories can live in the photos you choose to display in your home, the reminders you set on a shelf, and the silent rituals you practice. If you're not ready to put the story into words, try collecting objects that tell the story, and try to simply exist in their presence.

Audience

The audience problem is one of social dynamics. Some don't want to talk about their sibling *too* much for fear it will define them, especially in adolescence when no one wants to be known as the kid with the dead brother/sister. Others don't know whom to share these stories with, are cautious about other people's discomfort with the topic, or may feel pressure to keep them "in the family" due to stigma. In the same way you choose which stories to share, you also are in charge of your audience. Everyone you talk to doesn't need to get the same stories—or any story at all—but you can't only tell these stories to yourself. The true healing comes from your grief and pain being witnessed by another, and in the knowledge that your sibling's memory will live on in others.

Early in our conversation, Iestyn told me how much he enjoys talking about his twin brother, and that when the question of siblings comes up, he usually says he doesn't have any.

"Isn't that contradictory?" I asked. "You're saying both that you like talking about your brother, but also that you don't talk about him with people."

Iestyn then gave me a master class in nuance and owning our stories. What it comes down to, for him, is that he loves talking about the life he shared with his twin, not the way he left this world. When someone you just met learns you have a deceased sibling, the conversation most often goes to questions about the cause of death. So if that's not what you want to talk about, there's no easy way to skip over it and go straight to the good stuff. When Iestyn is around old friends and family, it's completely different because they can talk about his brother's life. When you own your story, you also own whom that story is told to and under what circumstances.

So what if there is no ideal audience? No one you'd trust with the new information and no one with whom to exchange the old? Then you need to make new friends. I'm sorry but it's true. The answer is not to repress the stories or bury them. Cara told me she tried, "but then I remember and I feel guilty." They will never stay buried. This is a completely new, life-altering experience for you, and that means you might not have people in your life who have experienced or are defined by this thing that has just rocketed you into a new reality. Good news is, there *are* people out there with similar experiences, and you can find them.

Here are just a few suggestions:

- **Al-Anon**—A mutual support program for people whose lives have been affected by someone else's drinking. https://al-anon.org
- **The Alliance of Hope**—Support groups, resources, and 24/7 online support forum for suicide loss survivors. allianceofhope.org
- **The American Foundation for Suicide Prevention**—Support groups and healing sessions for survivors of suicide loss. afsp.org
- **The Dinner Party**—A community for mourners in their twenties, thirties, and forties that fosters connection through a Grief Buddy or a seat at a virtual table with others experiencing loss. There are sibling-specific tables you can choose to join, as well as some that are based on cause of death, identity (BIPOC, LGBTQ+, etc.), or geography if you'd prefer to meet in person. https://www.thedinnerparty.org
- **The Dougy Center**—An online directory of local grief support groups for children, teens, and adults. Dougy also offers crisis support and resources. Dougy.org
- **Experience Camps**—A free one-week summer camp for children experiencing the loss of a parent, sibling, or primary caregiver. Camps are located across the US. experiencecamps.org
- **Nar-Anon**—A twelve-step program for family and friends of addicts. https://www.nar-anon.org
- **The National Alliance on Mental Illness (NAMI)**—An alliance of more than six hundred local organizations committed to educating, supporting, advocating, and improving the lives of people struggling with mental illness and their loved ones. NAMI offers virtual and in-person support groups for family members of people with mental health conditions. NAMI.org
- **The Tragedy Assistance Program for Survivors (TAPS)**—In-person and online support groups, 24/7 survivor helpline, programming, camps, and resources for those who have experienced a military loss, including survivors of military suicide. taps.org

- **What's Your Grief**—Resources, courses, and community for loss, including a platform to share your stories and photos and view others' stories. whatsyourgrief.com

If you're facing the audience obstacle, please do not let your stories melt away, I beg of you. Your stories matter. If they're not ready to see the light yet, that's okay, there are other ways you can preserve them until you find your deserving audience. Cara described writing as "a good way to talk about it without talking about it," and she's absolutely right. Writing, while overwhelming for some, is a profoundly safe space for others. Writing your stories is how you can best tell them to yourself, and that matters.

THE POWER OF STORY

Think about the value you get from hearing stories of other people who have been through loss. If you didn't find it valuable to hear about others' firsthand experiences, you wouldn't have made it this far in the book. Hearing stories normalizes the experiences, emotions, and realities that don't get talked about enough. Nearly 8 percent of Americans will lose a sibling before the age of twenty-five; you probably know someone who has lost a sibling and you don't even know it. You may be that person for someone else.

A few months ago, I was at a birthday party for a child in my son's class. My son asked me to stay, so I was one of the few parents lingering on the sidelines of their capture-the-flag game. I began chatting with another mother I'd met previously, and she asked what I did for a living. My husband had been encouraging me to talk about the book more, so I told her that I'm a researcher and am writing a book. It was a vague answer and bordered on a non-answer, but I'm working on it.

"What's the book about?" she asked.

"Oh, it's super depressing," I said with an awkward laugh. "It's about dealing with the loss of a sibling, sibling grief specifically. I'm still working on my elevator pitch."

"I'll read it when it comes out," she responded, smiling at me before looking away.

"That's very kind of you but I don't really expect everyone to read it."

"No, I really will read it," she insisted. "I should read it."

All nuance lost on me, I shrugged and said, "That's really nice of you, thanks."

"I'll read it because I'm your target audience. I lost my sister."

"Then you know," I said, looking her in the eyes, "there aren't a lot of resources for us. No one really talks about it."

She shook her head. "Losing my sister always felt like something that happened to my mom, not something that happened to me."

"That's really common," I told her. "That came up a lot in the interviews, and it's known to have caused things like delayed and complicated grief for the sibling."

Then the floodgates opened. She hadn't spoken to other people in her position, people who have lost siblings and are trying to navigate this new normal. She began asking me questions: "Have people talked about [insert topic that's come up over and over], or is that just me?" In response to each of her questions I was able to relay a different story, and they weren't just my stories. I was able to tell her the stories that are captured in this book, and those that go beyond it. Every few minutes she'd lean over and ask another question. She seemed increasingly curious about her own loss.

The conversation revived me. It reminded me why this book is so important and how much each of our stories can help others in the same position. When I recounted the story to my husband that night, riding high on the feeling of purpose and meaning, I passionately ranted, "She wasn't even able to feel ownership over her loss! She lost a sister! It happened to her parents, but it also happened to her! Who is looking out for her?!" Aaron listened intently and asked, "Have you reached out to her tonight? You may have just blown her world apart." I picked up my phone, realizing that, yes, that was definitely not the birthday party conversation she'd been expecting, and there was a text from her. Among other things, she wrote, "It was really nice to connect." That's what we did. Through our own stories and the stories of others we were able to connect, and each of us left feeling a little less alone, and a little more normalized.

One way to connect is by consuming the stories of others. Rob's mom gave him and his surviving siblings each a copy of Joan Didion's *The Year of Magical Thinking* after his sister's death. Ten years later, he found the forgotten book on a shelf and decided to (finally) read it. Rob describes the experience:

> Once I started I couldn't stop, and that's not me, I'm not that type of a reader. My wife would tell you that I can spend a year and get through one 250-page book. I would go to work, come home, put the kids to bed, and cruise up to my room, and I just plow through it. What spoke to me, and why it's too bad I waited way too long to read it, is that this book confirms so many of the wacky feelings that you feel when you are part of this lousy club. That book was really helpful to me even a decade later. It wasn't about sibling loss, but it was about loss, and it made me think "holy shit, I'm not batshit crazy." There are all sorts of crazy things that I thought about—continue to think about to some degree—that you don't have answers to, and there's no one to really reciprocate or bounce that off of in a comfortable way. At least there wasn't for me. To read what she wrote on paper was an affirmation that I am not in the loony bin, you know.

Here are some suggestions for stories on loss that may help you feel less alone. These are not all focused on sibling loss, but they all share the universal experience of grief:

- *Everything Is Horrible and Wonderful: A Tragicomic Memoir of Genius, Heroin, Love, and Loss*—Stephanie Wittels Wachs
- *The Year of Magical Thinking*—Joan Didion
- *Grief Is Love: Living with Loss*—Marisa Renee Lee
- *Modern Loss: Candid Conversation About Grief. Beginners Welcome*—by Rebecca Soffer and Gabrielle Birkner
- *The Catcher in the Rye*—J. D. Salinger
- *Notes on Grief*—Chimamanda Ngozi Adichie

- *It's OK That You're Not OK: Meeting Grief and Loss in a Culture That Doesn't Understand*—Megan Devine
- *It's Okay to Laugh: (Crying Is Cool Too)*—Nora McInerny
- *The Rules of Inheritance*—Claire Bidwell Smith
- *Crying in H Mart*—Michelle Zauner
- *I'm Glad My Mom Died*—Jennette McCurdy
- *Finding the Words: Working Through Profound Loss with Hope and Purpose*—Colin Campbell
- *Once More We Saw Stars*—Jayson Greene

fifteen

Legacy

If we ever leave a legacy, it's that we loved each other well.

—Indigo Girls

Ben thought about his legacy a lot more than I ever will. His journals are peppered with entries in which he explores the meaning of legacy and wonders what his own legacy will be.

August 22, 2000

Saturday morning I was napping out by the Iwo Jima memorial and listening to my "coming home from the road trip of '96" mix, and I heard "100 Years" by Blues Traveler for the first time in years. It used to be one of my favorite songs, and I know the lyrics had such a strong impact on my philosophies on life. But I'd forgotten about the song. I know I wrote about it in other journals, I'm curious to see what I thought back then. If I remember correctly, I don't want to be forgotten—I want to make a difference for the generation in one hundred years. At the same time, little things roll off my back so easily. Maybe it's part of my perspective that certain things matter and others don't matter as much. This will change—it has changed so much over the past few years. But I need to get back to the hundred-year focus. How will I make a difference in one hundred years?

Grandma Goldie made a difference that endures one hundred years later. She came to America, stowed away on a boat, and her choice—her initiative, bravery, intelligence led to Grandpa, who saved I don't know how many lives in WWII and Waterbury, then to Allen, Neal, Gary, and Jeff, then myself, Sam, Annie, all the cousins who have, I believe, made the world a better place. So Great-Grandma Goldie made a difference in one hundred years. What will I do?

Ben was an idealistic twenty-something, and as such these entries laid out grand plans with grand goals. That's a lot of pressure, for him and for us. I felt that pressure. It's why I nearly changed my entire life to pursue his dreams. I thought my job was to execute on the legacy he'd planned, which was impossible. I was paralyzed: If I can't execute his vision, do I have permission to create my own on his behalf?

I'm older now, a decade past my own idealistic twenties with two kids and a lot more perspective, and I've come to the conclusion that legacy doesn't need to be grand. After all, it was Ben's favorite band, Indigo Girls, who said, "If we ever leave a legacy, it's that we loved each other well." Reading Ben's entry again, I realize that, above all, our Great-Grandma Goldie's legacy is one of love. Her legacy is the love her family has for each other and humanity. And do you want to know the refrain, repeated over and over in Blues Traveler's "100 Years"?

And it won't mean a thing in a hundred years.

No, it won't mean a thing in a hundred years.

I wondered if Ben's fixation on legacy had impacted Sam's grief the same way it did mine, and if it was something he thought about or made a conscious effort at. So I did the thing that had become routine while writing this book: I texted him late on a Friday night with a half-baked question. "Do you ever think about Ben's legacy? Or do/keep/value things because of him?" He responded almost immediately, first with a joke (as is *his* routine) before telling me, "It, like, comes and goes. Thinking about him. Legacy. So it's there all the time I guess, but in the background. Like a song you love that comes on the radio every once in a while." I thanked him profusely and thought the conversation was over, until he replied again. "When Howard Stern recently interviewed Bruce Springsteen, I listened to the interview every day for a week and cried each time thinking about Ben. Which only makes sense to us, 'cause it's not like they ever talked about brothers. But that's when it hit me last I guess."

When I say I burst out crying, I mean I *burst* out. A sob was escaping before I'd even processed his whole message. I've been deep into sibling loss research for *years* at this point; I've now written an entire book on the significance of the loss and the fact that we never get over it. Why, then, was I so surprised when my brother told me he still cried about the loss? I had just assumed Sam was handling things better than me because his grief looked different from my own, but that wasn't fair to him or to me. I allowed myself to sit with that surprise and, as my therapist says, I "sent some curiosity" to it. It wasn't surprise—it was love. The image of my big brother listening to a podcast and crying about *his* big brother was as heart-wrenching as it was beautiful. The intimacy of it took my breath away and reminded me of a diary entry Ben had written after spending an evening with Sam in college:

Talked with the boy. There's something about brothers. Just the word— there's a bond, something shared which—I look up to him and he looks up to me. I'm sure Sam and I will be close forever.

Turns out he was right.

My son has been asking more and more questions about Ben. Not much about the details of his death, but about his life—and about how they are connected. When he was four, Archie asked if Ben was his brother.

"No, he was my brother," I responded.

"So what does that make him to me?" Archie asked, trying to puzzle together how this Ben character fits into our story.

"That makes him your uncle, just like Uncle Sam."

Understanding dawned on his face. "So I have two uncles?"

"Yes!" I exclaimed, inappropriate excitement in my voice.

His face fell. "I'm sad that I didn't know him," he said slowly, "but I'm glad he was my uncle."

As we hugged, I began to cry. (Obviously. I bet you're a little choked up yourself just reading this.) When we eventually pulled apart, Archie looked at my red-rimmed eyes and tear-streaked cheeks and said, "Mom, what's happening to your face right now?" And in that moment, I couldn't help but laugh because that's exactly what Ben would have said, and I knew he was right there with us trying to make things a little bit easier.

FINDING MEANING

Ben and I loved listening to *This American Life*. We'd always send each other great episodes we'd found in the archives, and we had an ongoing disagreement over which was the best episode ever (he thought it was "Babysitting," but I maintain it's "Music Lessons," in which David Sedaris sings commercial jingles in the voice of Billie Holiday). But I digress. A year or two after Ben's death, I thought about pitching his story—our story—to *This American Life*. What a great way to honor him, I thought; he'd get such a kick out of hearing Ira Glass say his name. I was excited about the idea except there was one minor issue—I had no idea how the story would end. *TAL* was looking for stories that had a clear beginning, middle, and end—that had a lesson and someone learned something. The stories had a meaning. I couldn't find the meaning; I just wanted to tell people all about my brother.

There's a lot of talk among grief researchers about the value of meaning-making in the aftermath of loss. I struggle with the word "meaning" myself; to me, "meaning" means that there was a reason this happened and that there is something productive or constructive to be done with the grief. That's a whole lot of pressure to put on a mourner. Now we need to figure out the meaning of life *and* the meaning of our loved one's death? No, thank you. But I've thought a lot about that theory—the idea that finding meaning in the death is what can truly bring healing—and I've slowly come around. I asked Stephanie Wittels Wachs about it, and whether her memoir about the year following her brother's death and the subsequent podcasts she's produced on addiction were her way of finding meaning. She was silent for a moment, leaning back as a hesitant smile crossed her face. Then she shook her head. "I've honestly never considered that." She seemed as surprised by her answer as I was. "I never thought of any of this as my way of finding meaning," she continued. "This is just survival." Throughout Wachs's work, one common thread is the unconditional love she has for her brother Harris. That unconditional love is, perhaps, the most essential meaning there is. What if instead of "finding meaning" we can find love?

I've come to believe that love is the ultimate legacy, and that love can come in all sorts of shapes and sizes. That type of legacy doesn't need to be grand, and it doesn't need to be public. Perhaps your loss taught you to give people the benefit of the doubt more readily because you realized everyone is fighting their own battle, even if you can't see it. Perhaps you're a little more kind; you make more of an effort to be a good friend; you tell your family how much you love them. No memorial plaques required.

LEGACY IN ACTION

In my research with bereaved siblings, their perceptions of "legacy" fell into six core themes. These are not mutually exclusive themes, and many explore different themes at different life stages. Some are more internal, with a focus on a continuing bond and an active presence in their life, while others focus the energy outward toward causes that their sibling was passionate about.

Stories

"I talk about him a lot with my kids. They need to understand that addiction is real, and I can use him as a vehicle for awareness and knowledge."

"He wanted to be seen and witnessed and heard, and no one was helping him. My job is to make sure people see him."

"My daughter has my brother's name as her middle name. It also happens to be my husband's name, so she talks about her name matching her papa, but also her name matches her uncle. That's an important reason for her own name. That's a piece of legacy right there, in the story of her name."

"I also do a yearly learning or taking on a kind deed around the day of her passing and send it to fifty to seventy-five of my friends. Most of them didn't know her, so I get to share about her and call them up to step up to their greatness in her honor."

Causes

"As my mental state got better, I could finally wrap my head around the fact that it was not my fault. Now through my work [as a therapist] I get to help other people understand that. I helped run a group for parents who suffered the death of a child, and we've even done a suicide loss retreat."

"These institutions of government, of society, truly failed in my circumstances. But the work that I've done as an adult in the space, what I have carved out for myself in my career, is working in these institutions in order to make them better to serve children and students. I work primarily in education and government, and have built a career out of forming better schools that are better for kids, but also that touch on all these other aspects that are supporting kids. And so part of me would be a resource provider, and actually making connections to create solutions, because that is what I do right now. And so the solutions didn't exist for me, and I've now built a career on creating those solutions to help kids."

"I think about him all the time and run a golf tournament in his honor. This summer will be the sixteenth year. We have raised probably $1.5 million to help kids in need attend camp."

"I feel like in order to honor her memory, and to leave a legacy, I needed to do something. There was never a question that I was going to be a domestic violence advocate."

Values

"He lives on in my conscious fostering of closeness amongst my own children. He lives on in the way I treasure my big sister, the one sibling I have now."

"My sister was incredibly empathetic and kind, and an incredible listener. She was excellent at being a human; checking in on you, asking how you are and empathizing with you. She was incredibly good at understanding your areas of concern, the pain points, and relating with you. It was genuine and it was authentic. . . . It was sort of a doubling down of just really basic human elements that I think we all forget about, but those were really important to her. When she was gone it became very apparent to me what was important to her, and how important those things are, too, to everyone. I try to emulate that as best I can, those things that she was so good at. When I talk about positives that have come from the loss, that's a real positive to me. Now that's totally separate from the fact that she killed herself. I would much prefer that she not. But I'm going to take that if it's one small, tiny lesson; I'm on it. And I'm going to hold on to that with much more weight than I hold on to anything relating to her taking her life."

"As long as I'm alive my brother is alive because he's alive in my brain and he is alive in my memories. He's alive in me, he's my twin brother, so he really is alive in me essentially."

Rituals and Traditions

"There are three traditions that our family and friends have, well, settled on I guess. The first is we all eat ice cream. Inevitably, on his birthday, we are all texting each other pictures of the ice cream we're eating (my brother loves chocolate ice cream). We all seem to have landed on a collective favorite color of orange. That's it, I guess that's not a tradition but it kind of is. And then we also have the postcards. It has tailed off some, but in those first few years the number of postcards that were sent were astounding. My brother Dan would say, 'Why do we send so many postcards? Because we buy too many postcards.' He was always writing postcards. So when he passed away, we picked it up."

"His life and his loss are a part of me. He is more than his death even though his death had a huge impact on my life alone. He lives on through his family and in his children. I am the main connector to his surviving children and to their Gwich'in heritage, and I remind them that through him they are connected to a tribe with a huge history that was important to my brother that they know. I have built ritual around his loss, and that has been helpful for me over the years."

"My daughter is only a baby, but I want to tell her about my brother and do things with her that I know he would have wanted to do with her."

"I write him a poem every year on his birthday, and then I do the same thing every year on the anniversary of his death. As I move a little bit further away from it, I get more comfortable with it, I guess. But on some level it's almost painful that this is my new normal. Right? Like, you get to this point where it's like, yeah, he's gone and I'm okay with it, but don't really want to be okay with it. So then you feel, like, bad about it?"

Projects

"My sisters and I were going to do a kid's [clothing] line using fabric from our home country and incorporate it into modern clothing. That's also when I realized that Nadine could actually draw because she started drawing the sketches and I thought, 'Oh, cool, okay. I did not know that about you.' But then when she got really, really sick, we had to put that aside. About four months after her passing I was organizing, and I found the sketches. She had named the lines already; I mean, she had really thought about this stuff. My [other] sister and I were like, okay, how about we try to do this. I see it as her legacy living on. I don't really see myself as someone who wants to be in the fashion business, per se, but it's something that we want to do."

"I continue to carry her legacy through sharing her story, the photographs and book I made of her memory. I am working on a book of the images I have from her life. As an artist I love that my work can carry on her story and share sibling love and the grief that comes with loss."

Physical Representations

"On the day I became older than he ever was, I got a tattoo on my wrist in memory of him. It's tiny and barely noticeable, but he loved things like that, and I've always hated tattoos, so I know it would make him really happy to see his little sister rebelling. Plus, it feels like I engraved a piece of him on me forever."

"I think about him almost every day and I keep a box of X-Men cards, bracelets, and notes he'd given me."

"A friend of mine who had lost her father had said to keep a bunch of his stuff. She said you're always gonna want more of his stuff. So I did. I grabbed random stuff, you know, and I still have it all. I have some T-shirts of his that I wear, and I have a pair of shoes of his that are a little too big, but I'll still wear them on occasion. I have a couple of his baseball hats I wear, and I also have a Patriots sweatshirt that I wear. The sweatshirt is one that I don't wear that often, but he's physically with me when I put that one on, you know what I mean? I know that I can feel him there."

These are just some of the ways we might integrate our siblings into our lives in such a way that allows us to incorporate the loss into our lives as we move forward. Looking back now (with the benefit of hindsight, therapy, and having written this book), I've realized that I held on to that acute grief for so long because I thought the only alternative was to move on and "get over it." I knew I'd never get over this. I couldn't imagine myself ever "getting over" my love for my brothers, so if the only way to heal was to stop loving, then I was destined to suffer forever. I didn't know there was room in between to incorporate our relationship in a positive way. I thought it was all or nothing.

By incorporating a variety of the above suggestions into my own life, I've been able to feel Ben's presence more. Our relationship feels alive again in a way I never thought possible, and I am no longer stuck in that complicated grief. I feel that love again but in a new way; I'm learning to love myself as unconditionally as he did. I've learned to fit my (very tall) brother into that hole in my heart and carry him with me.

Is it as good as when he was alive? No, of course not.

Do I still cry about the loss? As of writing this, it's been two hours since my last cry.

Would I give up all this perspective in exchange for getting him back? I sure would.

I can't get my brother back, but learning to carry that Polly Pocket–sized Ben doll in my heart is the next best thing.

THE END

Thirteen years after Ben's death I can report that I have found meaning—the love that remains—and I have certainly learned a lot, but I still don't know how my episode of *This American Life* ends. I don't know how this book will end either.

I wish I could tie it all up in a nice bow for you.

I wish I could tell you it all gets better and you'll be fine.

I wish I could assure you that this pain won't last.

I wish I could share a life-changing revelation that makes this all okay.

I wish I could give you your brothers and sisters back.

I wish I could be sandwiched in a hug by my own two big brothers.

This is all a consolation prize. It's an attempt to make lemonade out of rotten lemons, but I suppose that's the best we can do when rotten lemons are all we've got. I don't know how to end this book because grief, like love, never ends.

I might not be able to find the perfect ending, but I find myself wondering if Ben could. Throughout his journals, Ben returns again and again to the idea of writing a book. Sometimes he believes it to be a book about life, while other times his thoughts are more specific—a book about travel, about service. Each time, he explores the lessons he'd impart to you, his reader.

June 6, 2000

I've been wondering, tonight, if I were to become a writer, what I'd write about. It would have to be a collection of short essays, maybe letters. I write well in bursts, when I just write ideas, thoughts. I don't expand well, and I really don't enjoy or benefit from reading the expanded thoughts of others. I've been reading *Future Shock* by Alvin Toffler, which explains that if we look out at the past fifty thousand years, and assume that a lifetime lasts sixty-two years, we're on the eight hundredth lifetime. Of those eight hundred, 650 were spent living in caves, 158 were agrarian, two were industrial, and now we're in this post (super?) Industrial Age. Pretty clearly illustrates how time is literally speeding up. Also makes a point that for the first time, we can actually see, visualize, and understand the importance of our lives, how the speed of change makes us obsolete within one lifetime. Seems like a great reason to smile often (who said "you'd cry your eyes out if you didn't"—Indigo Girls). What chapters and essays could I write about?

- What it's like to be the kid stuck out in a group—crying because I was too tall. Being ditched at the beach. Hating kids you want to like you.
- The value of growing up outside the cool group, and still knowing you'd be okay. The advantages, the independence, the ability to venture outside the norm.
- Time alone, travel, disappearing, becoming someone new. Meeting new friends on a train. Traveling alone for days and losing your voice—losing the ability to communicate for lack of practice.
- The power of silence in a group. The value of silence. The power of invoking silence over a group.
- Faraway friends.
- Friends you see once a year and still hold an unmistakable, and perhaps insurmountable, power in my life.
- Determining a best friend. Do you need one? Was Mark my best friend? Was it Kevin?

- Falling asleep while talking, half conversations half dreams, responses, mixed lives.
- Mixing friendships. How to talk to all when you're a different person in each, do you try? Of course.
- The healing power of time, patience.
- Moving often, physically, emotionally. How easy it is, but how difficult it is to stay.
- Trust. Faith in others. Laughing. Keys to success in any group.
- Group dynamics. Growing together, leading together, learn comfort in authority, leadership, laughter. Hard times. Enjoying the experience.
- Riding the bus across America.
- Travel writing, voyages, trips home when I'm abroad.
- Family, love, confidence, keys to success and joy. Support and then some. Take the time.
- Taking care of others, taking care of friends. Listening, watching, supporting, laughing, encouraging, enjoying.
- Dedication—knowing—learning when to give up. Swimming crew. Taught to always do more, write the book report, play more, crying in the stands at swim practice and not knowing why. But also knowing why, and knowing I couldn't quit and wanted to win, but couldn't.

I'll go to sleep now with a slough full of memories all churned up and rolling inside.

—Ben S., June 6, 2000 (Annie's Sweet Sixteen),
11:00 p.m., Arlington Heights, Virginia

Exercises

These are here for you to use; cherry-pick, do them all, choose your own adventure . . . these are for you. Read them through and do the ones that feel good in that moment. These are for you and only you, so if they don't add comfort or support your grief, please skip them. You might come back to them at a later time—or not! It's important that your Mourner's User Manual is in a place/format where you can continually add to it and access it—that might look like a dedicated journal or notebook, or it could be notes on your phone, a folder on your laptop, or a huge roll of paper on your wall. Do what feels right, just do.

PART I: WITH (MINING FOR MEMORIES)

Chapter 2: Writing the Letter We'll Never Send

It's time to write your sibling a letter. Yes, I know your sibling died and does not currently have a mailing address; it's a letter you'll never send. Write with true and pure honesty about your relationship and the impact they had on your life, the good and the bad. However troubled or distant the relationship was, it was significant and so is this loss.

I won't make you start from a blank page (the horror!). To start, sit down with pen and paper and fill in the blanks:

- You always made me laugh when you _____.
- I could always get under your skin by _____.
- I hated it when you _____.
- I never told you that _____.
- I was furious at you when you _____
  because _____.
- I'm sorry that I _____.
- I always think of you when _____.
- If you were here right now, I'd tell you _____.
- I wish that _____.

Next, with your eyes closed, imagine your focus turning inside, and remind yourself that no one else ever needs to read this. Imagine your sibling is standing in front of you as you open your eyes, pick up a pen, and begin to write.

Dear _____ ,

Chapter 4: Memory Map

If you're like me, you might be preoccupied with the fear of forgetting those memories you hold dear. If so, and if you're ready, we can take a moment to begin collecting and preserving any memories you're afraid of forgetting.

1. Write your sibling's name in the center of a blank sheet of paper and draw a circle around it.
2. Surrounding their name, write the names of different phases or chapters of your life together. This could include things like early childhood, school, adolescence, college, summer camp, etc. Draw a circle around each one and draw a line connecting each individual circle to the circle in the center.
3. Choose one of those new circles and start writing memories from that chapter around it. You don't need to write the memories out in full, just one word to trigger your recollection is all it takes. Draw a circle around each new memory

and draw a line connecting each new individual circle to the life chapter.

4. Add more circles as you go, adding as many life chapters, memories, and memory offshoots as you can.

PART II: WITHOUT (MOURNER'S USER MANUAL)

Chapter 5: Mourner's User Manual: Operating Instructions

A really good user manual is able to explain complex issues (and solutions) to someone with zero relevant knowledge. It's my goal to help you gain the clarity and confidence needed to communicate your own unique needs to those around you in a way they will understand.

So let's get simple. Ultimately, my goal is to help you do this without overthinking. Please take as long (or short) as you want. Skip questions that don't feel good to you, and add your own information that I've forgotten. I like to do this quickly (to try to get ahead of that overthinking brain of mine), but you might want to go slower. This is a road map, but you should take this road at your own pace. Your answers to these questions, and the things that bring you calm, will change—sometimes by the day. Revisit this exercise as often as is helpful; nothing here is set in stone.

Step 1: At your own pace and in your own time, think through the following questions and, when helpful, note down the answers in your MUM:

- Do you find comfort in visiting the cemetery?
- Does it feel good to get outside and move your body?
- Does it feel good to talk to friends about your sibling?
- Are you angry?
- Do you feel guilt?
- Are you being honest with those around you?
- Do you know how to ask for help?
- Do your loved ones know how you feel?

- Imagine a friend drops off dinner—do you want them to come in and eat with you?
- What situations or environments help you feel calmer?
- When a friend texts and asks how you're doing, how do you feel?
- What are the most important things you want your friends to know?
- What are the most important things you want your family to know?

Step 2: Throughout the next week, write down every activity that brings you peace or calm. These activities may range from the ordinary (sleeping, showering) to the extraordinary (hiking in the woods, visiting a museum, screaming at the top of your lungs).

Step 3: At the end of the week, read through the list and write down the top three things that you will commit to doing on a regular basis moving forward.

Chapter 6: Facing Our Parents—Real or Imagined

You've written to your sibling, and now if it feels right, you can write a letter to your parents. If addressing your parents feels triggering or otherwise upsetting, this is a good one to skip and consider readdressing with the care and support of a mental health professional. If you do choose to proceed, you can write this with the intent of sharing with your parents or not. I've included prompts below to use as inspiration to get you started, but as always, they're optional.

- I am afraid to tell you that _____ because _____. If I did tell you, I'd hope that you would respond by _____ , but I'm afraid you would _____ instead.
- I want you to know that after _____ died, I felt _____. I didn't tell you at the time because _____.

- I wish you understood that _____.
- I wish I could help you _____.
- I wish you could help me _____.
- Before _____ died our family was
  _____ and now
  it's _____.
- I wish we could talk about _____, but I am
  afraid to bring it up because _____.

Chapter 7: Mourner's User Manual: Communication and Support

In this exercise we'll explore the types of support you do (and do not) find helpful. Remember, this need be for your eyes only. Don't worry about hurting anyone's feelings or adding qualifiers; as long as you're being honest, you're doing the right thing. The purpose of this exercise is to get some clarity for *yourself*, so only answer those that feel relevant and helpful:

- Do you like it when people come visit in person? What about talking on the phone or video calls?
- Do you prefer text messages or emails? Do you get any pleasure from responding to these messages, or does it feel like an obligation?
- If a friend comes by with food, do you want them to stay and eat with you or leave it outside your door?
- Is there anyone you can call if you need to talk in the middle of the night or the middle of the day?
- Is there anyone you call when you are most upset?
- Is there anyone you share stories and memories with?
- If you start crying in the middle of the day, is there a friend/colleague/classmate who can cover for you?
- Which TV show or movie makes you laugh through the tears? Which helps you cry big, cathartic tears?
- What food do you never want to see again? (I'm looking at you, Edible Arrangements.)

- What is the most helpful thing anyone has said to you during your time of mourning? What's the least helpful?
- If someone you know lost their sibling tomorrow, what would you tell them? How would you support them? How might you ask someone to support you in the same way?
- What do you wish you could ask of your friends and family? What is stopping you from asking?

Chapter 8: Outlets for Anger

Do you have your own version of the Ikea Dish Dance? Do you sometimes feel like your insides are going to burst but have no outlet, so you end up screaming at the asshole who cut the line in Java City without saying "excuse me"? Have you been holding in your anger this whole time, just waiting for the perfect inopportune moment for it to bubble over? We all hold and express anger differently, and we can sometimes (inadvertently) turn that anger on ourselves while we're busy acting "fine" for everyone else. I want you to give yourself permission to acknowledge and soothe that anger, no matter how "logical" or "unreasonable" it is. Whatever state your anger might be in, however far out from the loss you are, here are some prompts to help you identify a healthy outlet as you relinquish control and move through it.

1. Begin by sitting in a quiet, comfortable space and close your eyes. Think of your sibling—don't shy away. Try to see them in your mind with full clarity. Take note of where you feel the emotions in your body and focus on those areas.
   - What do those muscles *want* to do in this moment?
   - Where do you feel the most energy, pressure, pain?

2. Send some curiosity to those areas—do they need a physical release? Do they need a hug? Are they looking for permission to merely exist? What does that anger need in order to be released without denying it?

If your anger feels like it needs a *physical* release, think of activities that might help channel it. Does the idea of a boxing class sound good? What about soothing it with yoga or shaking it out with vigorous dance? Can you commit to trying one of the activities that feels right in your body?

If your anger lives more in your head and your heart, consider working it out on the page. The pen is mightier than the sword, after all. Allow yourself to breathe into the anger as you write down all the things you never allowed yourself to admit or express before. Are you angry at your sibling? Your parents? Friends whose siblings are alive and well? It doesn't matter how "unreasonable" the target—let your anger out onto the page without judgment.

Chapter 9: Soundtrack

If it's not clear by now, music gives me great solace. Maybe it can help you too. It's time to create a playlist that you can listen to when you need comfort, support, a good cry, or to feel the presence of your sibling. I've included my own "Ben's Ultimate Playlist" on pages 245–246; perhaps it will spark some inspiration.

All you need to do is identify one song, one single song that reminds you of your sibling. Doesn't matter if they ever even heard the song—it matters that you feel the relevance. Start with one.

Chapter 10: Answering Hard Questions

As you meet new people and enter into new relationships, the topic of siblings often comes up—as it should! Humans are curious beings. We build connections by learning about each other. I spent months terrified that someone would ask me how many siblings I have, and that I wouldn't know how to answer. That terror can make it difficult to build any connections at all.

I found it helpful to think about the different ways that question could be asked and how I could handle it, prepping myself before I was put on the spot. If you think that might help you too, below is a list of common questions I've gotten. Your answer will not be one-size-fits-all, and you can even answer differently every time if you want.

Remember, you do not owe anyone more than you are willing to give. A non-answer is perfectly acceptable.

Common questions:

1. How many siblings do you have?
2. Are they older? Younger? Brothers? Sisters?
3. Are you close with your sibling(s)?
4. Where do your sibling(s) live? What do they do?
5. How did they die? (If you've shared the loss.)

PART III: WITHIN (FACING THE FUTURE TOGETHER)

Chapter 11: Sharing the Good

In recent years I've found myself having more and more conversations with Ben in my head. I was always skeptical of people who said things like that, but now I am one and I get it. I get tremendous comfort from those small conversations, and I think you could too. Imagine your sibling is eager to catch up—free of judgment or jealousy. If you're not sure how to start, here are a few ideas:

- What is something that happened recently that you are proud of?
- What was the last thing that made you laugh?
- What new shows are you enjoying? Podcasts? Movies?
- Is there any celebrity news or gossip your sibling would enjoy?
- What's the most absurd thing you've seen on the internet this week?
- What's the most ridiculous thing someone has said to you recently?

Chapter 15: Embracing Legacy

Many of us do not know the full extent of our sibling's legacy, or what impact they had on those who knew them. If you are interested in learning more about the other facets of their life and feel it could help in your grief, then I encourage you to reach out beyond your immediate circle, connect with folks who knew your sibling, and listen to their stories.

Don't know where to start? That's okay. You can start anywhere you'd like. For some it might be easier to start with people you know well (that's what I did), and for others it will be easier to start with the most distant relationship first. Here are a few ideas of questions you might use as a jumping-off point:

- How would you describe your relationship with _____ ?
- Tell me about them . . . how would you describe them to someone who never met them?
- What's your first memory of them?
- What's your best memory of them?
- What did they mean to you?
- What has been the hardest part about losing them?
- What would you ask or tell _____ if they were here today?
- How do you think they'd want to be remembered?
- Is there something about _____ that you think no one else knows?
- How are you different now than you were before you lost _____ ?

If possible, I recommend recording these conversations for posterity. You're going to want to focus on the conversation itself as it's happening, not on taking notes or making sure you captured each detail. A recording allows you to revisit the conversation on your own time and terms.

Acknowledgments

First, to the people who made this book possible in the most literal sense. Thank you to the 350 bereaved siblings who took the time out of their day to fill out a survey about one of the worst things that ever happened to them. You didn't know me, you had no reason to trust me, and yet you did. And to the brave souls who agreed to follow-up interviews and gamely answered all my questions; LN, SK, RF, RK, RA, AE, SS, RL, KG, KJ, SA, CE, AB, SR, CL, KH, JS, CM, SSC, JG, BB, CO, MS: this book would not exist without you, your stories, and your siblings. Thank you for sharing them with all of us.

To my agent, Eryn Kalavsky, thank you for telling me you'd take me on as a client only if I was willing to tell my own story, instead of hiding in the margins. Eryn, I am so grateful to you for making me an author.

To Renee Sedliar, my dream editor. I never dared hope that I would find an editor who was such a perfect fit for what I needed *and* was a member of this club, and then I met you. I hate that you know far too well what it's like to lose a sibling. Thank you for going on this journey with me, encouraging me, and reminding me why we all need this book.

To my dear friends and fellow club members who acted as sounding boards, researchers, and experts. Beth Newell, I don't think I would've gotten through this process without our weekends together. Thank you for always letting me talk about the worst things that ever happened to us, for your honesty, and for your years-long quest to help me see the signs. Beth, you have given me my brother back, and for that there are no words to thank you. Jennifer Jackson, I am forever grateful for the time, dedication, and care you poured into helping me bring this together from start to finish, research through final read.

To the Pile and Loss x3, you let me think aloud through many late nights and early ideas, you opened up about your own losses and fears, and you reinforced this vague idea I had that we all need this book. Thank you to Samara, Anna, Kate, Elizabeth, Stephanie, Jessica, Jess, and all the other Pilers for believing in me, encouraging me, and helping me have fun along the way.

To Hanna Stein and Lynn Casey, my professional mentors, personal idols, and friends. Thank you for making me a better researcher by constantly reminding me of the humanity, empathy, and curiosity that drive us all forward. And to David Dunbar, who taught me the magic of questions.

To Kevin, Jeff, Joe, and Boyar, the gentlemen, my surrogate big brothers, my friends. Thank you for your openness. I know it wasn't easy when I reached out ten years later looking to reopen wounds; thank you for allowing us all to heal together.

To Lissa, my sister in every way except blood (and height). I treasure your friendship and am eternally grateful that you were waiting on the kitchen counter when my parents brought me home from the hospital. Thank you for supporting me, encouraging me, and reminding me that Ben's memory and legacy live on beyond the confines of our nuclear family. He was like a brother to you, and he loved you so much.

Thank you to my friends; my incredible lifesaving, joke-making friends who have become family, and my family who have become friends. Thank you for sitting with me in silence when I had no words but couldn't be alone. Thank you for understanding when I'd disappear and for welcoming me when I climbed back.

To Wendi, Redmond, Edie, Ben, and Goldie; thank you for infusing life and joy into our family. I always envisioned my kids having a large extended family and when Ben died, I was afraid that future died with him. You all proved me so wrong, and I couldn't be happier about it. I am proud to say that I am one of us.

To Sam (in case you've read this far), thank you for putting yourself out there and allowing me to constantly trigger and retrigger your grief via middle-of-the-day texts and random phone calls asking you about the worst moment of our lives. You believed in me from the very beginning, and I really needed that.

Mom and Dad, from the moment we lost Ben, you have been there for me in my grief, and I have never questioned your support, not for a moment. Thank you for validating and acknowledging the magnitude of my loss and allowing us each to grieve in our own way. Our family didn't crumble after Ben died; because of you, we grew closer and stronger. Thank you for the gift of our family.

To my kids, Archie and Mazie (and Gilda): I'm not sure what to call the special kind of magic you both possess, but it's magic all the same. You knew when I needed cheering up and cheering on, you told me I could do this, and you told me you were proud of me. You two (three) fill my bucket beyond overflowing each and every day. I'm so lucky to be your mom and to be a recipient of your magic; I hope I can continue to make you proud. I love you, unconditionally.

And finally, to Aaron. Instead of fumbling for words that could never truly encompass all that you mean to me, I'm going to close my laptop, wrap my arms around you, and never let go. Got a sec? I love you.

Bibliography

Barrera, Maru, Rifat Alam, Norma Mammone D'Agostino, David B. Nicholas, and Gerald Schneiderman. "Parental Perceptions of Siblings' Grieving After a Childhood Cancer Death: A Longitudinal Study." *Death Studies* 37, no. 1 (2013): 25–46. https://doi.org/10.1080/07481187.2012.678262.

Bladek, Marta. "'A Place None of Us Know Until We Reach It': Mapping Grief and Memory in Joan Didion's *The Year of Magical Thinking*." *Biography* 37, no. 4 (2014): 935–952. https://doi.org/10.1353/bio.2014.0059.

Bonanno, George A. *The Other Side of Sadness: What the New Science of Bereavement Tells Us About Life After Loss*. New York: Basic Books, 2019.

Borchet, Judyta, Aleksandra Lewandowska-Walter, Piotr Połomski, Aleksandra Peplińska, and Lisa M. Hooper. "We Are in This Together: Retrospective Parentification, Sibling Relationships, and Self-Esteem." *Journal of Child and Family Studies* 29, no. 10 (2020): 2982–2991. https://doi.org/10.1007/s10826-020-01723-3.

Brach, Tara. *Radical Acceptance: Embracing Your Life with the Heart of a Buddha*. New York: Bantam Books, 2004.

Brewster, Annie. *The Healing Power of Story: The Art and Science of How Sharing Your Personal Story Can Improve Your Health*. Avon, MA: Adams Media Corporation, 2020.

Brown, Brené. *Atlas of the Heart: Mapping Meaningful Connection and the Language of Human Experience*. New York: Random House, 2021.

Campione-Barr, Nicole, and Sarah E. Killoren. "Love Them and Hate Them: The Developmental Appropriateness of Ambivalence in the Adolescent Sibling Relationship." *Child Development Perspectives* 13, no. 4 (2019): 221–226. https://doi.org/10.1111/cdep.12345.

Cohen, Orit, and Michael Katz. "Grief and Growth of Bereaved Siblings as Related to Attachment Style and Flexibility." *Death Studies* 39, no. 3 (2015): 158–164. https://doi.org/10.1080/07481187.2014.923069.

Cooper, Anderson. *Stephen Colbert and Anderson Cooper's Beautiful Conversation About Grief*. CNN, 2019. https://www.youtube.com/watch?v=YB46h1koicQ.

Currier, Joseph M., Jason M. Holland, and Robert A. Neimeyer. "Sense-Making, Grief, and the Experience of Violent Loss: Toward a Mediational Model." *Death Studies* 30, no. 5 (2006): 403–428. https://doi.org/10.1080/07481180600614351.

Currier, Joseph M., Jennifer E. Irish, Robert A. Neimeyer, and Joshua D. Foster. "Attachment, Continuing Bonds, and Complicated Grief Following Violent Loss: Testing a Moderated Model." *Death Studies* 39, no. 4 (2014): 201–210. https://doi.org /10.1080/07481187.2014.975869.

Davies, Katherine. "Siblings, Stories and the Self: The Sociological Significance of Young People's Sibling Relationships." *Sociology* 49, no. 4 (2014): 679–695. https://doi .org/10.1177/0038038514551091.

DeVita-Raeburn, Elizabeth. *The Empty Room: Surviving the Loss of a Sister or Brother at Any Age.* New York: Scribner, 2004.

Dickens, Nancy. "Prevalence of Complicated Grief and Posttraumatic Stress Disorder in Children and Adolescents Following Sibling Death." *The Family Journal* 22, no. 1 (2013): 119–126. https://doi.org/10.1177/1066480713505066.

Didion, Joan. *The Year of Magical Thinking.* HarperCollins UK, 2021.

Ephron, Delia. *Sister Mother Husband Dog (Etc.).* New York: Penguin Group USA, 2013.

Fletcher, Jason, Marsha Mailick, Jieun Song, and Barbara Wolfe. "A Sibling Death in the Family: Common and Consequential." *Demography* 50, no. 3 (2012): 803–826. https://doi.org/10.1007/s13524-012-0162-4.

Frances Taylor, Myra, Nadia Clark, and Elaine Newton. "Counselling Australian Baby Boomers: Examining the Loss and Grief Issues Facing Aging Distance-Separated Sibling Dyads." *British Journal of Guidance & Counselling* 36, no. 2 (2008): 189–204. https://doi.org/10.1080/03069880801926442.

Funk, Amy M., Sheryl Jenkins, Kim Schafer Astroth, Gregory Braswell, and Cindy Kerber. "A Narrative Analysis of Sibling Grief." *Journal of Loss and Trauma* 23, no. 1 (2017): 1–14. https://doi.org/10.1080/15325024.2017.1396281.

Gillette, Hope. "What Are the Types of Grief?" Psych Central, December 19, 2022. https://psychcentral.com/health/types-of-grief.

Gillies, James, and Robert A. Neimeyer. "Loss, Grief, and the Search for Significance: Toward a Model of Meaning Reconstruction in Bereavement." *Journal of Constructivist Psychology* 19, no. 1 (2006): 31–65. https://doi.org/10.1080/10720530500311182.

Goodman, Susan. "Traumatic Loss and Developmental Interruption in Adolescence: An Integrative Approach." *Journal of Infant, Child, and Adolescent Psychotherapy* 12, no. 2 (2013): 72–83. https://doi.org/10.1080/15289168.2013.791150.

Gungordu, Nahide, Maria Hernandez-Reif, Youn-Jeng Choi, and David-Ian Walker. "The Reliability and Validity of the Lifespan Sibling Relationship Scale (LSRS) with an English-Speaking Young Adult Sample." *Families in Society: The Journal of Contemporary Social Services* 102, no. 4 (2021): 548–555. https://doi .org/10.1177/1044389421992289.

Herberman Mash, Holly B., Carol S. Fullerton, and Robert J. Ursano. "Complicated Grief and Bereavement in Young Adults Following Close Friend and Sibling Loss." *Depression and Anxiety* 30, no. 12 (2013): 1202–1210. https://doi.org/10.1002 /da.22068.

Hill, Tatiana Yasmeen, and Natalia Palacios. "Older Sibling Contribution to Younger Children's Working Memory and Cognitive Flexibility." *Social Development* 29, no. 1 (2019): 57–72. https://doi.org/10.1111/sode.12400.

Holinger, Dorothy P. *The Anatomy of Grief.* New Haven: Yale University Press, 2020.

Hyatt, Erica Goldblatt. "Shifting Identities, Shifting Meanings: Adolescent Siblings and Grief." In *Narrating Practice with Children and Adolescents*, edited by Mery F. Diaz and Benjamin Shepard, 298–312 (New York: Columbia University Press, 2019). https://doi.org/10.7312/diaz18478-018.

Jackson, Laura Lynne. *Signs: The Secret Language of the Universe.* New York: Random House, 2020.

Kelly, Liz. "16 Different Types of Grief." Talkspace, November 20, 2022. https://www.talkspace.com/blog/types-of-grief/.

Kempson, Diane, and Vicki Murdock. "Memory Keepers: A Narrative Study on Siblings Never Known." *Death Studies* 34, no. 8 (2010): 738–756. https://doi.org/10.1080/07481181003765402.

Kessler, David. *Finding Meaning: The Sixth Stage of Grief.* New York: Scribner, 2020.

Kluger, Jeffrey. *The Sibling Effect: What the Bonds Among Brothers and Sisters Reveal About Us.* New York: Riverhead Books, 2012.

Kübler-Ross, Elisabeth. *On Death and Dying: Questions and Answers on Death and Dying: On Life After Death.* New York: Quality Paperback Book Club, 2002.

Kübler-Ross, Elisabeth. *On Grief and Grieving.* New York: Scribner, 2005.

Kukla, Elliot. "It's Okay to Forgive, or Not: Grieving When You're Estranged from Your Family." The Body Is Not an Apology, August 3, 2021. https://thebodyisnotanapology.com/magazine/when-theres-no-hollywood-ending-how-do-i-grieve-the-dying-when-i-am-estranged-from-family/.

Lee, Marisa Renee. *Grief Is Love: Living with Loss.* New York: Legacy Lit, 2023.

McHale, Susan M., Kimberly A. Updegraff, and Shawn D. Whiteman. "Sibling Relationships and Influences in Childhood and Adolescence." *Journal of Marriage and Family* 74, no. 5 (2012): 913–930. https://doi.org/10.1111/j.1741-3737.2012.01011.x.

Merino, Laura, Ana Martínez-Pampliega, and David Herrero-Fernández. "A Pilot Study of Younger Sibling Adaptation: Contributions of Individual Variables, Daily Stress, Interparental Conflict and Older Sibling's Variables." *Europe's Journal of Psychology* 17, no. 2 (2021): 1–12. https://doi.org/10.5964/ejop.2139.

Neimeyer, Robert A. "Meaning Reconstruction in Bereavement: Development of a Research Program." *Death Studies* 43, no. 2 (2019): 79–91. https://doi.org/10.1080/07481187.2018.1456620.

Neimeyer, Robert A. "Searching for the Meaning of Meaning: Grief Therapy and the Process of Reconstruction." *Death Studies* 24, no. 6 (2000): 541–558. https://doi.org/10.1080/07481180050121480.

Neimeyer, Robert A., Anna Laurie, Tara Mehta, Heather Hardison, and Joseph M. Currier. "Lessons of Loss: Meaning-Making in Bereaved College Students." *New Directions for Student Services*, no. 121 (2008): 27–39. https://doi.org/10.1002/ss.264.

Neimeyer, Robert A., Carlos Torres, and Douglas C. Smith. "The Virtual Dream: Rewriting Stories of Loss and Grief." *Death Studies* 35, no. 7 (2011): 646–672. https://doi.org/10.1080/07481187.2011.570596.

Neimeyer, Robert A., Scott A. Baldwin, and James Gillies. "Continuing Bonds and Reconstructing Meaning: Mitigating Complications in Bereavement." *Death Studies* 30, no. 8 (2006): 715–738. https://doi.org/10.1080/07481180600848322.

Opelt, Amanda Held. *Hole in the World: Finding Hope in Rituals of Grief and Healing.* New York: Worthy Publishing, 2023.

Packman, Wendy, Heidi Horsley, Betty Davies, and Robin Kramer. "Sibling Bereavement and Continuing Bonds." *Death Studies* 30, no. 9 (2006): 817–841. https://doi.org/10.1080/07481180600886603.

Paris, Megan M., Brian L. Carter, Susan X. Day, and Mary W. Armsworth. "Grief and Trauma in Children After the Death of a Sibling." *Journal of Child & Adolescent Trauma* 2, no. 2 (2009): 71–80. https://doi.org/10.1080/19361520902861913.

Rasouli, Omid, Unni Karin Moksnes, Trude Reinfjell, Odin Hjemdal, and Mary-Elizabeth Bradley Eilertsen. "Impact of Resilience and Social Support on Long-Term Grief in Cancer-Bereaved Siblings: An Exploratory Study." *BMC Palliative Care* 21, no. 1 (2022). https://doi.org/10.1186/s12904-022-00978-5.

Rolbiecki, Abigail J., Karla T. Washington, and Katina Bitsicas. "Digital Storytelling as an Intervention for Bereaved Family Members." Omega, March 2021. https://www.ncbi.nlm.nih.gov/pmc/articles/PMC7819462/.

Sedaris, David. "Now We Are Five." *New Yorker*, October 21, 2013. https://www.newyorker.com/magazine/2013/10/28/now-we-are-five.

Shepherd, Daniel, Sonja Goedeke, Jason Landon, Steve Taylor, and Jade Williams. "The Impact of Sibling Relationships on Later-Life Psychological and Subjective Well-Being." *Journal of Adult Development* 28, no. 1 (2020): 76–86. https://doi.org/10.1007/s10804-020-09350-4.

Silverman, Gila S. "Saying Kaddish: Meaning-Making and Continuing Bonds in American Jewish Mourning Ritual." *Death Studies* 45, no. 1 (2020): 19–28. https://doi.org/10.1080/07481187.2020.1851887.

Skagerberg, Elin M., and Daniel B. Wright. "Sibling Differentials in Power and Memory Conformity." *Scandinavian Journal of Psychology* 50, no. 2 (2009): 101–107. https://doi.org/10.1111/j.1467-9450.2008.00693.x.

Smith, Claire Bidwell. *Anxiety, the Missing Stage of Grief: A Revolutionary Approach to Understanding and Healing the Impact of Loss.* New York: Hachette Go, 2020.

Soffer, Rebecca, and Gabrielle Birkner. *Modern Loss: Candid Conversation About Grief. Beginners Welcome.* New York: Harper Wave, 2018.

Sveen, Josefin, Alexandra Eilegård, Gunnar Steineck, and Ulrika Kreicbergs. "They Still Grieve—a Nationwide Follow-up of Young Adults 2–9 Years After Losing a Sibling to Cancer." *Psycho-Oncology* 23, no. 6 (2013): 658–664. https://doi.org/10.1002/pon.3463.

Tidwell, Brandy L., Elizabeth D. Larson, and Jacob A. Bentley. "Attachment Security and Continuing Bonds: The Mediating Role of Meaning-Made in Bereavement." *Journal of Loss and Trauma* 26, no. 2 (2020): 116–133. https://doi.org/10.1080/15325024.2020.1753389.

Wiking, Meik. *The Art of Making Memories: How to Create and Remember Happy Moments.* New York: William Morrow, 2019.

Williams, Honey, Jordan Skalisky, Thane M. Erickson, and John Thoburn. "Posttraumatic Growth in the Context of Grief: Testing the Mindfulness-to-Meaning Theory." *Journal of Loss and Trauma* 26, no. 7 (2020): 611–623. https://doi.org/10.1080/15325024.2020.1855048.

Wolfelt, Alan. *Healing the Adult Sibling's Grieving Heart: 100 Practical Ideas After Your Brother or Sister Dies*. Fort Collins: Companion Press, 2008.

Wray, T. J. *Surviving the Death of a Sibling: Living Through Grief When an Adult Brother or Sister Dies*. New York: Three Rivers Press, 2003.

Zak, Paul J. "How Stories Change the Brain." Greater Good Magazine, December 17, 2013. https://greatergood.berkeley.edu/article/item/how_stories_change_brain.

Notes

Introduction

1. Kübler-Ross, Elizabeth and David Kessler. *On Grief and Grieving*. New York: Scribner, 2005.

2. Brown, Brené. *Rising Strong*. New York: Spiegel & Grau, 2015.

Chapter 1

1. Funk, Amy M., Sheryl Jenkins, Kim Schafer Astroth, Gregory Braswell, and Cindy Kerber. "A Narrative Analysis of Sibling Grief." *Journal of Loss and Trauma* 23, no. 1 (2017): 1–14. https://doi.org/10.1080/15325024.2017.1396281.

Chapter 2

1. Shepherd, Daniel, Sonja Goedeke, Jason Landon, Steve Taylor, and Jade Williams. "The Impact of Sibling Relationships on Later-Life Psychological and Subjective Well-Being." *Journal of Adult Development* 28, no. 1 (2020): 76–86. https://doi.org/10.1007/s10804-020-09350-4.

2. Kluger, Jeffrey. *The Sibling Effect: What the Bonds Among Brothers and Sisters Reveal About Us*. New York: Riverhead Books, 2012, 10.

3. Packman, Wendy, Heidi Horsley, Betty Davies, and Robin Kramer. "Sibling Bereavement and Continuing Bonds." *Death Studies* 30, no. 9 (2006): 817–841. https://doi.org/10.1080/07481180600886603.

4. Kluger, Jeffrey. *The Sibling Effect: What the Bonds Among Brothers and Sisters Reveal About Us*. New York: Riverhead Books, 2012, 6.

5. Shepherd, Daniel, Sonja Goedeke, Jason Landon, Steve Taylor, and Jade Williams. "The Impact of Sibling Relationships on Later-Life Psychological and Subjective Well-Being." *Journal of Adult Development* 28, no. 1 (2020): 76–86. https://doi.org/10.1007/s10804-020-09350-4.

6. Kluger, Jeffrey. *The Sibling Effect: What the Bonds Among Brothers and Sisters Reveal About Us*. New York: Riverhead Books, 2012, 40.

7. McHale, Susan M., Kimberly A. Updegraff, and Shawn D. Whiteman. "Sibling Relationships and Influences in Childhood and Adolescence." *Journal of Marriage*

and Family 74, no. 5 (2012): 913–930. https://doi.org/10.1111/j.1741-3737.2012 .01011.x.

8. Funk, Amy M., Sheryl Jenkins, Kim Schafer Astroth, Gregory Braswell, and Cindy Kerber. "A Narrative Analysis of Sibling Grief." *Journal of Loss and Trauma* 23, no. 1 (2017): 1–14. https://doi.org/10.1080/15325024.2017.1396281.

9. Herberman Mash, Holly B., Carol S. Fullerton, and Robert J. Ursano. "Complicated Grief and Bereavement in Young Adults Following Close Friend and Sibling Loss." *Depression and Anxiety* 30, no. 12 (2013): 1202–1210. https://doi.org/10.1002 /da.22068.

Chapter 3

1. Soffer, Rebecca, and Gabrielle Birkner. *Modern Loss: Candid Conversation About Grief: Beginners Welcome.* New York: Harper Wave, 2018, 309.

2. Ephron, Delia. *Sister Mother Husband Dog (Etc.).* New York: Penguin Group USA, 2013, 10.

3. "The 'Forgotten Bereaved': Grief over Losing an Adult Sibling May Go Unacknowledged." *The Harvard Mental Health Letter* 25, no. 3 (2008): 6.

4. Kübler-Ross, Elisabeth. *On Death and Dying: Questions and Answers on Death and Dying: On Life After Death.* New York: Quality Paperback Book Club, 2002.

5. Soffer, Rebecca, and Gabrielle Birkner. *Modern Loss: Candid Conversation About Grief. Beginners Welcome.* New York: Harper Wave, 2018, 137–145.

6. Smith, Claire Bidwell. *Anxiety: The Missing Stage of Grief: A Revolutionary Approach to Understanding and Healing the Impact of Loss.* New York: Hachette Go, 2020, 89.

Chapter 4

1. Wiking, Meik. *The Art of Making Memories: How to Create and Remember Happy Moments.* New York: William Morrow, 2019, 8.

2. Ibid.

3. Skagerberg, Elin M., and Daniel B. Wright. "Sibling Differentials in Power and Memory Conformity." *Scandinavian Journal of Psychology* 50, no. 2 (2009): 101–107. https://doi.org/10.1111/j.1467-9450.2008.00693.x.

4. Wiking, Meik. *The Art of Making Memories: How to Create and Remember Happy Moments.* New York: William Morrow, 2019, 8.

5. Brown, Brené. *Atlas of the Heart: Mapping Meaningful Connection and the Language of Human Experience.* New York: Random House, 2021, 77.

6. Bonanno, George A. *The Other Side of Sadness: What the New Science of Bereavement Tells Us About Life After Loss.* New York: Basic Books, 2019, 71.

7. Ibid.

8. Ibid.

9. Wiking, Meik. *The Art of Making Memories: How to Create and Remember Happy Moments.* New York: William Morrow, 2019, 11.

10. Kempson, Diane, and Vicki Murdock. "Memory Keepers: A Narrative Study on Siblings Never Known." *Death Studies* 34, no. 8 (2010): 738–756. https:// doi.org/10.1080/07481181003765402.

Chapter 5

1. Kelly, Liz. "16 Different Types of Grief." Talkspace, November 20, 2022. https://www.talkspace.com/blog/types-of-grief/.

2. Gillette, Hope. "What Are the Types of Grief?" Psych Central, December 19, 2022. https://psychcentral.com/health/types-of-grief.

3. Herberman Mash, Holly B., Carol S. Fullerton, and Robert J. Ursano. "Complicated Grief and Bereavement in Young Adults Following Close Friend and Sibling Loss." *Depression and Anxiety* 30, no. 12 (2013): 1202–1210. https://doi.org/10.1002/da.22068.

4. Ibid.

5. Holinger, Dorothy P. *The Anatomy of Grief.* New Haven: Yale University Press, 2020, 39.

6. Herberman Mash, Holly B., Carol S. Fullerton, and Robert J. Ursano. "Complicated Grief and Bereavement in Young Adults Following Close Friend and Sibling Loss." *Depression and Anxiety* 30, no. 12 (2013): 1202–1210. https://doi.org/10.1002/da.22068.

7. Zampitella, Christina. "Adult Surviving Siblings: The Disenfranchised Grievers." *Group* 35, no. 4 (2011): 333–347. http://www.jstor.org/stable/41719337.

8. Moffa, Gina. *Moving on Doesn't Mean Letting Go: A Modern Guide to Navigating Loss.* New York: Balance, 2023.

9. Ibid.

10. Holinger, Dorothy P. *The Anatomy of Grief.* New Haven: Yale University Press, 2020.

11. Goodman, Susan. "Traumatic Loss and Developmental Interruption in Adolescence: An Integrative Approach." *Journal of Infant, Child, and Adolescent Psychotherapy* 12, no. 2 (2013): 72–83. https://doi.org/10.1080/15289168.2013.791150.

12. Dickens, Nancy. "Prevalence of Complicated Grief and Posttraumatic Stress Disorder in Children and Adolescents Following Sibling Death." *The Family Journal* 22, no. 1 (2013): 119–126. https://doi.org/10.1177/1066480713505066.

13. Packman, Wendy, Heidi Horsley, Betty Davies, and Robin Kramer. "Sibling Bereavement and Continuing Bonds." *Death Studies* 30, no. 9 (2006): 817–841. https://doi.org/10.1080/07481180600886603.

14. Buckley T., D. Sunari, A. Marshall, R. Bartrop, S. McKinley, and G. Tofler. "Physiological Correlates of Bereavement and the Impact of Bereavement Interventions." *Dialogues in Clinical Neuroscience* 14, no. 2 (2012): 129–139. doi: 10.31887/DCNS.2012.14.2/tbuckley. PMID: 22754285; PMCID: PMC3384441.

15. Holinger, Dorothy P. *The Anatomy of Grief.* New Haven: Yale University Press, 2020, 127.

16. Ibid., 135.

Chapter 6

1. Packman, Wendy, Heidi Horsley, Betty Davies, and Robin Kramer. "Sibling Bereavement and Continuing Bonds." *Death Studies* 30, no. 9 (2006): 817–841. https://doi.org/10.1080/07481180600886603.

2. Funk, Amy M., Sheryl Jenkins, Kim Schafer Astroth, Gregory Braswell, and Cindy Kerber. "A Narrative Analysis of Sibling Grief." *Journal of Loss and Trauma* 23, no. 1 (2017): 1–14. https://doi.org/10.1080/15325024.2017.1396281.

3. Packman, Wendy, Heidi Horsley, Betty Davies, and Robin Kramer. "Sibling Bereavement and Continuing Bonds." *Death Studies* 30, no. 9 (2006): 817–841. https:// doi.org/10.1080/07481180600886603.

4. Dickens, Nancy. "Prevalence of Complicated Grief and Posttraumatic Stress Disorder in Children and Adolescents Following Sibling Death." *The Family Journal* 22, no. 1 (2013): 119–126. https://doi.org/10.1177/106648071350 5066.

5. Funk, Amy M., Sheryl Jenkins, Kim Schafer Astroth, Gregory Braswell, and Cindy Kerber. "A Narrative Analysis of Sibling Grief." *Journal of Loss and Trauma* 23, no. 1 (2017): 1–14. https://doi.org/10.1080/15325024.2017.13 96281.

Chapter 7

1. Funk, Amy M., Sheryl Jenkins, Kim Schafer Astroth, Gregory Braswell, and Cindy Kerber. "A Narrative Analysis of Sibling Grief." *Journal of Loss and Trauma* 23, no. 1 (2017): 1–14. https://doi.org/10.1080/15325024.2017.1396281.

2. Sveen, Josefin, Alexandra Eilegård, Gunnar Steineck, and Ulrika Kreicbergs. "They Still Grieve—a Nationwide Follow-Up of Young Adults 2–9 Years After Losing a Sibling to Cancer." *Psycho-Oncology* 23, no. 6 (2013): 658–64. https://doi.org/10 .1002/pon.3463.

Chapter 8

1. Sveen, Josefin, Alexandra Eilegård, Gunnar Steineck, and Ulrika Kreicbergs. "They Still Grieve—a Nationwide Follow-Up of Young Adults 2–9 Years After Losing a Sibling to Cancer." *Psycho-Oncology* 23, no. 6 (2013): 658–664. https://doi.org/10.1002 /pon.3463.

2. Packman, Wendy, Heidi Horsley, Betty Davies, and Robin Kramer. "Sibling Bereavement and Continuing Bonds." *Death Studies* 30, no. 9 (2006): 817–841. https:// doi.org/10.1080/07481180600886603.

3. Fletcher, Jason, Marsha Mailick, Jieun Song, and Barbara Wolfe. "A Sibling Death in the Family: Common and Consequential." *Demography* 50, no. 3 (2012): 803–826. https://doi.org/10.1007/s13524-012-0162-4.

4. Herberman Mash, Holly B., Carol S. Fullerton, and Robert J. Ursano. "Complicated Grief and Bereavement in Young Adults Following Close Friend and Sibling Loss." *Depression and Anxiety* 30, no. 12 (2013): 1202–1210. https://doi.org/10.1002 /da.22068.

Chapter 9

1. Herberman Mash, Holly B., Carol S. Fullerton, and Robert J. Ursano. "Complicated Grief and Bereavement in Young Adults Following Close Friend and Sibling

Loss." *Depression and Anxiety* 30, no. 12 (2013): 1202–1210. https://doi.org/10.1002/da.22068.

2. Brown, Brené. *Atlas of the Heart: Mapping Meaningful Connection and the Language of Human Experience.* New York: Random House, 2021, 88.

3. Ibid.

4. "The 'Forgotten Bereaved': Grief over Losing an Adult Sibling May Go Unacknowledged." *Harvard Mental Health Letter* 25, no. 3 (2008): 6.

Chapter 10

1. Dickens, Nancy. "Prevalence of Complicated Grief and Posttraumatic Stress Disorder in Children and Adolescents Following Sibling Death." *The Family Journal* 22, no. 1 (2013): 119–126. https://doi.org/10.1177/1066480713505066.

2. Cohen, Orit, and Michael Katz. "Grief and Growth of Bereaved Siblings as Related to Attachment Style and Flexibility." *Death Studies* 39, no. 3 (2015): 158–164. https://doi.org/10.1080/07481187.2014.923069.

3. Maldenbert, Michelle P. "The Healing Power of Radical Acceptance." *Psychology Today*, March 3, 2022. https://www.dropbox.com/scl/fo/nnige5csrkuqjzketqz0m/h?rlkey=5haimgvhxxk5atgqiixm0b306&dl=0.

4. Brach, Tara. *Radical Acceptance: Embracing Your Life with the Heart of a Buddha.* New York: Bantam Books, 2004.

Chapter 11

1. Brown, Brené. *Atlas of the Heart: Mapping Meaningful Connection and the Language of Human Experience.* New York: Random House, 2021, 215.

2. Kukla, Elliot. "It's Okay to Forgive, or Not: Grieving When You're Estranged from Your Family." The Body Is Not an Apology, August 3, 2021. https://thebodyisnotanapology.com/magazine/when-theres-no-hollywood-ending-how-do-i-grieve-the-dying-when-i-am-estranged-from-family/.

3. Cooper, Anderson. *Stephen Colbert and Anderson Cooper's Beautiful Conversation About Grief.* CNN, 2019. https://www.youtube.com/watch?v=YB46h1koicQ.

Chapter 12

1. Packman, Wendy, Heidi Horsley, Betty Davies, and Robin Kramer. "Sibling Bereavement and Continuing Bonds." *Death Studies* 30, no. 9 (2006): 817–841. https://doi.org/10.1080/07481180600886603.

2. Sedaris, David. "Now We Are Five." *New Yorker*, October 21, 2013. https://www.newyorker.com/magazine/2013/10/28/now-we-are-five.

Chapter 13

1. Packman, Wendy, Heidi Horsley, Betty Davies, and Robin Kramer. "Sibling Bereavement and Continuing Bonds." *Death Studies* 30, no. 9 (2006): 817–841. https://doi.org/10.1080/07481180600886603.

2. Ibid.

Chapter 14

1. Zak, Paul J. "How Stories Change the Brain." *Greater Good Magazine*, December 17, 2013. https://greatergood.berkeley.edu/article/item/how_stories_change_brain.

2. Brewster, Annie. *The Healing Power of Storytelling: The Art and Science of How Sharing Your Story Can Improve Your Health*. Avon, MA: Adams Media Corporation, 2020, 43.

3. Rolbiecki, Abigail J., Karla T. Washington, and Katina Bitsicas. "Digital Storytelling as an Intervention for Bereaved Family Members." Omega, March 2021. https://www.ncbi.nlm.nih.gov/pmc/articles/PMC7819462/.

Ben's Ultimate Playlist

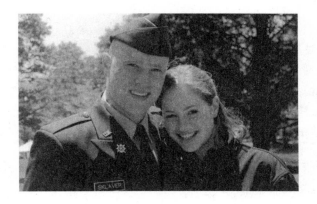

VOLUME 1

1. For a Dancer–Jackson Browne
2. My Sister–Juliana Hatfield
3. Unconditional I (Lookout Kid)–Arcade Fire
4. Murder in the City–The Avett Brothers
5. Hand Me Downs–Indigo Girls
6. Fake Empire–The National
7. Miles Away–Marc Cohn
8. Strangers–The Kinks
9. Head Full of Doubt–The Avett Brothers
10. Moonshadow–Yusuf / Cat Stevens
11. Talking Union–Woody Guthrie
12. Do You Realize?–The Flaming Lips
13. Without You–Eddie Vedder
14. Run-Around–Blues Traveler
15. Don't Stop Believin'–Journey
16. Green Grass & High Tides–The Outlaws
17. Hero–Family of the Year
18. As Cool as I Am–Dar Williams
19. Power of Two–Indigo Girls

VOLUME 2

1. Walkabout–Blue States
2. Wake Up–Arcade Fire
3. Wide Open Spaces–The Chicks
4. 100 Years–Blues Traveler
5. What a Good Boy–Barenaked Ladies
6. Closer to Fine–Indigo Girls
7. Cold Missouri Waters–Cry Cry Cry
8. Waiting Room–Fugazi
9. You Never Can Tell–Chuck Berry
10. Ring of Fire–Johnny Cash
11. Nightswimming–R.E.M.
12. Don't Think Twice, It's All Right–Bob Dylan
13. The Weight–The Band

Index

About the Author

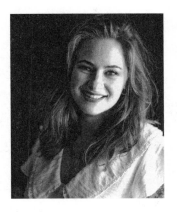

Annie Sklaver Orenstein is a qualitative researcher, oral historian, and storyteller who has spent over a decade collecting stories from people around the world on behalf of companies including Google, Viacom, Mattel, Instagram, Facebook, Pfizer, Netflix, Johnson & Johnson, and more. Her work has been featured on *NBC Nightly News*, Comedy Central, HuffPost, *Politico*, *TIME*, and Mother.ly. In 2020, driven by a desire to share these stories beyond the walls of corporate America, Annie founded Dispatch from Daybreak, a collection of letters written by womxn to their earlier selves. She lives in Connecticut with her husband, children, dog, and chickens.